DEATH, DYING AND RESIDENTIAL CARE

To my children, my sister and my grandmother
and
in memory of my mother and father.

Death, Dying and Residential Care

YVONNE SHEMMINGS

Avebury

Aldershot • Brookfield USA • Hong Kong • Singapore • Sydney

Published by
Avebury
Ashgate Publishing Limited
Gower House
Croft Road
Aldershot
Hants GU11 3HR
England

Ashgate Publishing Company
Old Post Road
Brookfield
Vermont 05036
USA

British Library Cataloguing in Publication Data

Shemmings, Yvonne
    Death, dying and residential care
    1. Death 2. Aged - Institutional care
    I. Title
    362.6'1

ISBN 1 85972 431 0

Library of Congress Catalog Card Number: 96-84606

Printed and bound by Athenaeum Press, Ltd.,
Gateshead, Tyne & Wear.

Contents

v

Acknowledgements

My gratitude goes to all those who participated in the research, in particular for the way they talked to me so candidly about their professional and personal experiences concerning death and dying; but it is the residents with whom I had contact, and the staff caring for them, who inspired me to conduct this research and who helped me to ask the right questions.

The research which forms the basis of this book was undertaken between 1993 and 1995 as part of my research master's thesis at the University of East Anglia, Norwich. Consequently my appreciation is also extended to Professor David Howe, Professor Martin Davies and Dr. Liz Trinder for their academic rigour, and to Ann MacDonald for her tutorial guidance and sensitivity. Finally I would like to thank my husband David for his emotional support.

Introduction

Mary is a young care assistant. Three years ago she returned home and found her fiancé dead, lying in bed. He had taken an overdose of his medication, prescribed for depression. In her job, Mary has to cope with her feelings when she hears people in their eighties and nineties crying with pain, saying that they want to die, or listen to people distressed and lost in their confusion. She says she seeks peace in the faces of residents when they have died to help lay to rest the ghost of her contorted fiancé. She is afraid that death is always distressing and full of pain. She likes to tend to residents immediately after they have died to make sure that their relatives may see them looking peaceful.

Mary was one of the twenty residential carers working in Homes for older people who were interviewed as part of this qualitative research study into the experiences of staff caring for residents during the later stages of life.

Not everyone faced such stark tragedies but, nevertheless, among the twenty, many had a touching story to tell about their personal experiences. One worker lost her mother to cancer when she was nineteen and had seen the distressing results of the post-mortem examination; one worker described her distress on discovering that her mother had committed suicide at the very time she had been telephoning her to arrange a reunion after many years of silence following a family rift; another worker's daughter has a rare, life-threatening brain disease; one has a seriously disabled husband who is completely dependant upon her. Yet another cares for a friend with multiple sclerosis.

For others the pressures were different. Alice walks down the corridor in answer to the sound of a buzzer from the lounge. John wanted to go to the toilet but was unable to wait. His clothes need changing. There are others too who need help to go to the toilet. It is almost lunch-time and there are people who need wheeling to the dining-room, before the food gets cold: if the Inspectors or the Environmental Health Officer make an unannounced call a report will be sent to senior managers if the food has fallen below a certain

1

temperature. A relative is waiting to see how his mother is . . . and all the while Jane is dying, alone, in her room.

This is part of the context in which residential carers for older people spend their working life. Being a manager of such staff it had struck me for some time that older people living and dying in local authority residential care seem not to be afforded the same consideration and sympathy as younger people dying in other institutions such as hospices; nor do staff experience the level of training offered in more specialist institutions. Perhaps it is simply that younger people cut down in their prime are missed and mourned more than older people, who may be felt to have 'outstayed their welcome'; or as Hughes put it in a recent publication:

> The assumption may be that because older people are closer to death and should therefore expect losses of various kinds, the impact when it occurs is less intense, less acute and less traumatic than with younger people. (Hughes, 1995, p. 123).

Naturally, matters concerning life and death are never simple and it is the inevitable complexity of death and dying which this book seeks to explore.

Many people do not experience the death of a friend or relative until quite late in their lives; for others death is an integral part of their experience of life, and in particular their working lives. Unlike the mourning protocols of the Victorians, or those within the traditions of some religions (for example within Judaism), in modern secular society the ritual of mourning has all but vanished. Furthermore, as society expects the 'show to go on', then this cultural expectation impinges upon the micro-culture of residential care. As a result staff experience death and dying around them in socially constructed terms. Unfortunately, as Habermas reminds us,

> Culture is unable to provide convincing answers to . . . existential questions like the quality of life in old age, the unity and integrity of the life cycle, and the meaning of ageing. (Habermas, 1974, cited in Longman, 1987).

The following extracts from Field and James (1993) contain interesting statistics about where older people tend to end their days:

> By the mid-1960s, two thirds of all deaths in the United Kingdom occurred in hospitals or other places caring for the sick, and by 1989 this had risen to 71% with only 23% of home deaths (p. 8) . . . Currently, 12-15% of all deaths occur in residential and nursing homes, *a figure that is likely to rise* (emphasis mine). Field and James, 1993, p. 17).

2

This rise in provision is also partly a reflection of a growing elderly population and an acknowledgement that, as the birth rate continues to fall in the United Kingdom, the responsibility for paying for care ultimately will fall on fewer people in the future. Increasingly too, carers of frail older people are in paid employment and to date there has been little recognition by employers of the stress placed on employees caring for elderly relatives (Phillips, 1994).

But who are the recipients of residential care for older people, and who are the staff who work in it? To appreciate the context of the book it is necessary to consider these questions. In recognising that people prefer to remain in their own homes the National Health and Community Care Act, 1990 arguably has been instrumental in attempting to ensure that only the most frail and needy enter residential care. In a study of dependency in residential care between 1980 and 1982 Booth (1985, p. 219) argued that 'contrary to general opinion, there is no sign of a continuing upward trend in levels of dependency' and that high rates of mortality and a steady flow of permanent transfers to hospital relieve old people's homes of many of their more severely dependant residents. However, Cartwright (1991) claims that 'the evidence suggests that because of their age and frailty those living in residential homes will have needed more care during the last year of their lives than other people who died' (p. 634). Furthermore - and of direct relevance to the present study - she concludes: 'Increasingly, the quality of life during the year before death is going to depend on the attributes of residential homes and their staff' (p. 627). She challenges Booth's earlier findings and suggests that, far from admission to hospital relieving residential homes from the care of the dying, it is possible that those living in residential homes are less likely than 'others who have died to have gone into a hospital or hospice during the last year of their lives or to die in one' (Cartwright, 1991).

The book is in three parts. Part One consists of a critical review of the relevant literature. Part Two presents the findings of a qualitative research study based upon the experiences of staff who regularly provide care to people in residential homes during the later stages of life. Finally, Part Three discusses some of the tensions and dilemmas emerging from the study, especially as they relate to care practice with older people who are dying.

Part One
REVIEW OF THE LITERATURE

'For what is it to die but to stand naked in the wind and to melt in the sun? And what is it to cease breathing but to free the breath from its restless tides, that it may rise and expand and seek God unencumbered?'

Kahlil Gibran

1 Death and dying

Medical events and social constructions

A recent publication produced by Counsel and Care (1995) included the following comment:

> There is very little literature and even less research on this theme. Though death is more readily discussed, very little has been written on death and dying within residential and nursing home settings. (Counsel and Care, 1995, p. 8).

Even less appears in the literature which refers directly to the experiences of those caring for people dying in institutions. Although a great deal of literature exists about death and dying generally, little empirical research has been conducted in the United Kingdom on the subject (Walter, 1992). When studies have been undertaken they have been carried out largely from the perspective of medical sociology (e.g. Williams, 1989), and in particular within the hospital setting (see, for example, Field, 1989 and Perakyla, 1988). As stated already, and of particular relevance to the present study, 'very little has been written on death and dying in residential and nursing home settings (Care and Counsel, 1995).

According to Bond and Bond (1994) over the last fifty years three main changes are apparent in the way death has been studied. Firstly, notions of 'mortality', 'disease' and 'causation' have been replaced with concerns about 'attitudes', 'sentiments' and 'awareness'. Secondly, researchers have become more interested in the perceptions of those involved in death and dying - the professionals, the bereaved, and those who die - (Davitz and Davitz, 1975). Thirdly, there has been an interest shown in the 'expressed wish to die' (see Dewey et al, 1993) and euthanasia. Indeed, it is this more 'human' side of

7

death and dying which gave rise to the hospice movement and the development of bereavement counselling (Dickenson and Johnson, 1993).

In short there is more attention paid to the social construction of death and dying. Bond and Bond (1994) argue that death in modern Western society is a lonely event, a process linked to the rise of individualisation. Referring to the work of Benoliel (1978) and De Vries (1981) they also conclude that others view death as 'bureaucratised, medicalised and hospitalised, to such an extent that it has been de-humanised' (p.171). Similarly Prior (1989) concluded that a number of changes have taken place during this period of time, each of which affects the way society understands and then organises death.

A congruence is detectable within the literature that death is not a simple biological event and that dying is not a diagnosis but a *predictive* term suggesting that the event of death will occur both within a medically and socially defined period of time - what Glaser and Strauss (1965b) called the 'dying trajectory'. Also, Bond and Bond (1994), find that the literature is unequivocal about the extent to which social behaviour in Britain stresses the living rather than the dying or the dead (and see Marris, 1974) as evidenced by the reduction in mourning rituals, the move towards 'secular rather than religious funerals (and the) increase in cremation over burial, (and) high remarriage rates among the younger widowed' (p.189).

Death has also been studied anthropologically (see, for example, Radcliffe-Brown, 1922). Rosenblatt (1983) concluded that mourning rituals contained features associated with *rites de passage* and Gorer (1965) was one of the first to argue that when such customs were abandoned it was the first sign of the 'denial of death' in Western culture (see Kellehear, 1989). Of particular relevance to this research were the findings from Prior's study of death notices. He found that those who were very old and had suffered from dementia, as well as elderly single women of no known occupation, tended to be under-represented (Prior, 1989).

Finally, Carse (1980, p. vii) identified ten ways in which death has been explained by philosophers, each of which reflects the way that faith, culture and personal beliefs influence attitudes towards death. He concluded that death was seen as a process of *change* by Plato. Modern science on the other hand - and perhaps as expected - links death with mere *dispersion* and *disregard* (whereas Freud and the psychoanalysts took a different view consistent with the unconsciousness of significant parts of human existence). Jung and the analytical psychoanalysts considered death as a *threshold*. Hinduism sees death as an *illusion*, with all things being reborn into the cosmos, albeit in an altered state; whereas in Christianity death is seen as *transformation* and is linked to faith in the risen Christ. Judaism, on the other hand, views death as an *inevitability*. According to Carse, some existential philosophers wrote of death

8

as *possibility* and therefore as a means of power. Finally, others see death as *horizon* and *discourse*: the metaphor of death is a distant event, yet which can be understood by human actors.

Perception and images of mortality: taboo ... or not taboo?

Metaphors of death and dying

When Socrates was on trial for his life, apparently he said 'No-one knows with regard to death whether it is not really the greatest blessing that can happen to man; but people dread it as though they were certain that it is the greatest evil...' This dilemma is reflected in the literature too: for some people, the word death strikes horror into the heart, yet for others it is something to be embraced, to be welcomed as a blessed relief. But for many the idea of death is taboo, not to be spoken about, not to be acknowledged (Hinton, 1972); yet equally this notion often has been challenged by anthropologists (see Fortune, 1932, for example) and other writers (Thomson, 1991; Kearl, 1989; Blauner, 1966 in Walter, 1992).

Unsurprisingly perhaps, there is little agreement as to what death *means* to individuals but a general assumption exists that, if people cannot die at home with their loved ones around them, then they seem to prefer to die surrounded by professionals in some sort of medical setting (Ariès, 1981). That individuals prefer to die in this setting appears to result from society's fear of death and the family's reluctance to care physically for relatives (Ariès, 1981). But Ariès goes on to argue that this may be where *society prefers* its citizens to die, away from the public gaze, where death makes it feel uncomfortable. It is argued further by some that death may have been stripped of its impact: even though it is given considerable exposure in the media, the reality remains distant from society. By shifting the experience of caring for the dying from the family (see Pincus, 1974) and placing the duty on institutions, traditional rituals may have been eroded.

Seale (1995), however, is highly critical of the notion that death is a taboo subject, or is routinely 'denied'. He criticises Gorer (1965), Armstrong (1987), Elias (1985) and, in particular, Ariès (1981). He also takes issue with the more recent argument in social theory that death is 'sequestered' from public space, citing Mellor (1993) and Shilling (1993) as being erroneous in their assumptions. Seale's objection is expressed thus,

In fact, calls to cease denying death and to resist 'medicalisation' have not gone unheard. Within the hospice movement psychological expertise is

9

marshalled to ensure that death is anticipated, prepared for, and above all accompanied. (Seale, 1995, p. 377).

Recently he has conducted research into the experiences of 149 relatives, friends and others who knew people who had died *alone*. One of his findings was that,

> Thus, when people die alone, ostensibly failures of emotional accompaniment, others engage in retrospective attempts to repair an order that has been damaged. This paper argues that the provision of an account of the death is an opportunity for resurrective practice. (p. 378).

He concludes thus,

> The hospital is a key site for the placement of death . . . and placement of the dying in institutions is a practice that can be understood as contributing to what Elias (1985) has called the 'civilising process', whereby the violent and 'animalic' aspects of human life - defecation, urination, sex or suffering - are restrained and pacified. The maintenance of emotional order and the regulation of the dying trajectory in hospitals is well documented. In this sense, placement of death in hospital is a response to the threat of disorder posed by allowing this event to occur elsewhere. This pacifying and regulatory effect is what has come to be criticised by those who bemoan the 'denial of death', associating this with its 'hiding away' in hospitals . . . However, a death in hospital, or a life in an institution, can also come to be understood as a disorderly threat to the ideals of the caring community. (pp. 389-390).

For Seale, the crux of the matter is that 'hospitals appear not to offer opportunities for *accompaniment*' (p. 390, emphasis mine). Far from the community being seen as *denying* death, Seale believes that its members are at pains to 'resurrect the last moments of the person who died, and claim membership of a caring community' (p. 388).

Naturally, society does not wish to be reminded constantly of its own inevitable mortality. In a culture where health, wealth, intelligence and activity are highly valued, and where the sick, infirm, old and disabled are marginalised (Thompson, 1993), it is of supreme importance to individuals that they are not seen to 'give in' to death and disease. Individuals within the culture strive to stay healthy, active and involved in the milieu of *life*. But, it is claimed that the *reasons* for not talking about death have changed over the centuries. Ariès (1974) concluded that the contemporary era of tabooed death arose, in part, from the attempts of those close to the sick and dying person to conceal their condition (in order to spare their feelings). The patient on the other hand in effect becomes responsible for the management of his or her own stigma (Goffman, 1964) and then also has to take care that the efforts of the others to ease matters are seen as effective and appreciated. Ariès developed this point further, suggesting that an interpersonal dynamic between the living and the dying - ' . . . the disturbance and the overly strong and unbearable emotion caused by the ugliness of dying and by the very presence of death in the midst of a happy life' (Ariès, 1974) - became culturally accepted and that the denial of death followed.

But, if death is in some way denied in modern western culture it appears that the fear of death and its denial have not always been the norm. Despite an alleged taboo surrounding death today, for centuries it inspired passion and creativity (Koestler, 1977) and, as we have seen already, it has always been the subject of philosophical consideration much of which concludes that part of the essence of life is to make sense of its ultimate end.

Although it is suggested that 'in itself death is nothing' (Carse, 1980) its presence regularly haunts us, possibly *because* it is beyond our comprehension; but human beings have always had different ways of making sense of their ultimate demise:

> People tend to die as they have lived as suggested by the saying 'Death is terrible to Cicero, desirable to Cato and indifferent to Socrates'. (Zarit, 1978, p. 265).

Although in some respects the idea of death nowadays has become repugnant and feared, if the word had been absent from our vocabulary 'our great works of literature would have remained unwritten, pyramids and cathedrals would not exist, nor works of religious art . . . '(Koestler, 1977, p. 52).

Along with Ariès (1981), Gorer (1965) argues that, as with sex, death is a powerful example of the way in which nature threatens culture. Blauner (1966), however, contends that death in modern society is *not* taboo, rather it is simply 'no big deal'. He believes it is *not* forbidden, merely hidden and, to some extent, Ariès (1981) would appear to concur with this idea. After all death is all around us; there is rarely a newspaper or news report on the television which does not have an item describing some form of death. For example, the National Institute of Mental Health identified that 'by the age of sixteen, the typical American has witnessed some eighteen thousand homicides on television in different guises' (Kearl, 1989, p. 383). Not only does a day rarely pass without at least one newspaper discussing death, bereavement, hospices or funerals, the literature is multiplying, as evidenced in Simpson's 1979 English language bibliography - which listed over 650 books on the subject - while his 1987 update adds another 1,700 books produced between 1979 and 1986 (Walter, 1992).

Thus the media has a profound influence on how death is viewed (Kearl, 1989). It is suggested by Gorer (1965) that there is a saturation of images of death in the media. He described this as the 'pornography of death'. But even though images of death are brought daily to us, commentators argue that there remains a tension between fiction, as experienced through films, magazines and books, and reality, as experienced by those who work directly with dying people, whether in an institution, through accidents, war or natural disaster.

Death postponed and delayed

It is argued within the literature that, not only has there been a change in the way society treats the subject of death (leading to its consequent professionalisation) since the mid-nineteenth century, but also there has been a change in focus upon who dies (Kearl, 1989). Then the interest was on people dying before what was considered their allotted time - their 'three score years and ten'. People are now living beyond this time. In the literature this is termed 'post-mature death' (to distinguish it from 'pre-mature' death). What is more 'there has been a shift in the focus of the death ethos from premature to postmature death' (Kearl, 1989). This could have implications for how death is perceived both at a macro-societal level and at a micro-level within the institutions which manage the death process, and for the ways in which health care workers and others cope with death and dying (Davitz and Davitz, 1975; Shanfield, 1981).

There is a growing movement which seeks to gain control over the death process. Ariès (1981) emphasised the importance of control, and introduced the idea of the 'good' death - one which was controlled - by contrasting it with the 'bad' death - the one for which we are unprepared. He identified a cultural need for those who are dying to be prepared for death, thus enabling a 'good' death to follow:

> Instead of an *Ars Moriendi* for coping with externally caused, premature death, and uncontrollable deaths, there has arisen the 'death with dignity' movement with recipes for personal control over 'on time', controllable deaths. (Ariès, 1981).

But the idea of preparation for death is not a new one. Sikhs, like Christians - and indeed many other faiths - talk about the concept of a 'good death'. They share a belief that what constitutes a 'good' death is the degree to which there

12

is a meditative period of time preceding it. Such a death 'does not take one unawares' (Ariès, 1981, p. 76). In the seventeenth century dying 'well' meant total vigilance, being prepared to meet one's 'maker': 'Death was fearful, courage was essential and victory was the prize' (Houlbrooke, 1989, p. 16).

In the light of this analysis, nowadays death-bed scenes are becoming a thing of the past: 'loving partings and solemn last words are gone'. More and more, the dying ' . . . are now sedated, comatose, manipulated and subconscious, if not sub-human' (Ariès, 1981). This somewhat bleak view of the end of life is echoed by Kearl (1989) who stated that in 'a society that views this world as the net totality of existence and in a desire to break from Christian tradition, death has become an alien intruder, disrupting the satisfactions of the here and now' (Kearl, 1989, p. 194).

So, as death is around us, how true is it that death is taboo? It may be that an element of implied narcissism persists: death happens to someone *else*. If a taboo does exist perhaps its roots lie in such a denial. Consequently, it may be tempting - and certainly less threatening - to view death from 'the outside', to feel sorry for the other person. The result leads to confusion, both at an individual and at a societal level. On the one hand 'A heavy silence has fallen over the subject of death' (Littlewood, 1992) yet on the other, it seems there is an ever-increasing need to know more about death. Nevertheless, nowadays the passage from life to death largely goes unnoticed by society and is marked by minimal ritual:

> Except for the death of statesmen, society has banished death. In towns, there is no way of knowing that something has happened; the old black and silver hearse has become an ordinary grey limousine, indistinguishable from the flow of traffic. Society no longer observes a pause; the disappearance of an individual no longer affects its continuity. Everything in town goes on as if nobody died any more. (Littlewood, 1992).

Whilst Lofland (1978), for example, acknowledges an increasing interest in matters concerning death there is little evidence that this is a change which goes beyond the voyeuristic or the personal (Ariès, 1981). Thus, according to Lofland (1978), disease has become an adversary; something to be 'fought', something against which to marshal 'courage'. The regular assertion that death is taboo fulfils this function by metaphorically evoking an enemy, which may explain partially why the taboo seems to persist even though more people talk about death. Furthermore, although it is now fashionable for some to talk more frankly about death, there is no convincing evidence to suggest that society wishes to return the act of death to the family.

To complicate matters even further, it is possible that the taboo surrounding death is not common to everyone: 'The limited taboo thesis argues that it is not modern society per se, but particular key occupational groups within it that find death peculiarly difficult to handle' (Lofland, 1978). It is recognised that caring for the dying is a major cause of stress for nurses and doctors (Vachon, 1987; Payne and Firth-Cozens, 1987). Thus, it is possible that it is the very people who experience the rawness of death firsthand who are the ones for whom a taboo continues to exist (but such a conclusion may overlook the possibility that an unwillingness to talk about death may differ with respect to residents, and with other colleagues for example). If this were the case, then inevitably a tension would exist between its development at a cultural and societal level, compared to within the micro-society of the institution where the sick and 'the old are sent to die' (Kearl, 1989). And if so, the sanitisation of death would enable it to be taken away from society's experience:

. . . When people want their dying to be put in hospitals, it is only partly because they hope for treatment which will save them. In reality it is because we can't face death. (Kearl, 1989).

2 Ageing, death and dying

Historical and cultural perceptions of ageing

People now live longer than ever before. In the period between 1817-31 life expectancy in Britain was 40 years for males and 42 years for females (Victor, 1987). By the mid-twentieth century the age at death changed from being distributed evenly across all age groups to that of occurring predominantly among old people: it changed from 'relative randomness' to 'predictability' (Cole, 1992). In 1986 79 per cent of those who died were 65 and over and 55 per cent were 75 and over (OPCS, 1989).

This demographic trend is having a significant impact both on the way old age is viewed by society, and on the care needed by the very old. While Seale (1991) argues that old age is not necessarily perceived as a terminal state he concludes that the problems of the older population have much in common with the problems of the dying.

From the literature it is possible to conclude that Western society has grown to accept elderly people provided they remain fit, healthy, active and still fighting. According to Zarit (1978), the earliest known Western text that relates to old age is by Ptah-hotep, an ancient Egyptian philosopher and poet, who wrote in 2500 BC:

> How hard and painful are the last days of an aged man! He grows weaker every day; his eyes become dim, his ears deaf; his strength fades; his heart knows peace no longer; his mouth falls silent and he speaks no word. The power of his mind lessens and today he cannot remember what yesterday was like. All his bones hurt. Those things which not long ago were done with pleasure are painful now; and taste vanishes. Old age is the worst of misfortunes which can afflict a man. (Zarit, 1978, in Victor, 1987, p. 72).

This somewhat gloomy description of the weakness and pain of old age was also reflected in the writings of Victorian moralists and social reformers (e.g. Shaftsbury, Wilberforce etc.) who divided the last stage of life into two apparently separate and controllable parts: the 'good' old age - of virtue, health, self-reliance, natural death and salvation; and the 'bad' old age - of sin, disease, dependency, premature death, and damnation (Cole, 1992).

But these ideas were not exclusive to the Victorians. Most ancient Egyptians, it seems, saw old age as a burden, both for the individual and society (Victor, 1987) and it is this view which has been more prevalent since the late nineteenth century, when the fear of old age and the possibility of a denial of death in society generally became infused with ideological and political meaning (Longman, 1987; Becker, 1973). In the late nineteenth century in America, for example, old age 'came to symbolise an intractable barrier to the dream of limitless accumulation of health and wealth' (Longman, 1987, p. 235).

Negative societal views towards the aged in Western culture are not new (although this is not the case in every culture). In Israel and China there tends to be more respect accorded to the aged, as a result of a cultural link having been forged between age and wisdom. Ancient Jews saw age as the ultimate reward for virtue. Consequently elderly people achieved considerable political power (Victor, 1987).

Social utility and the control of death

We have seen that human-beings may have a need to rationalise their experience of death and dying in a wish for satisfactory 'endings' and a desire to *control* death. According to Butler (1963) members of contemporary society have much in common with their ancestors during the last century:

> Impelled by their perfectionism in physical and spiritual matters and by their belief in the power of the individual will, Victorian moralists dichotomised and rationalised experience in order to control it. Ideological and psychological pressures to master old age generated a dualism that retains much of its cultural power today. (Butler, 1963, p. 422).

In an analysis of 'natural' and 'good' deaths in the seventeenth century Beier (1989) found that 'natural' deaths (such as death in childbirth and in old age) were not necessarily regarded as 'good', because they lacked the essential element of human control (Beier, 1989, p. 78). Smith (1905) reflects in his writing the Victorian proposition that to achieve a good old age it is essential to maintain health and usefulness to society, the notion highlighted by, among

16

others, Townsend (1964) and Phillipson and Walker (1986) as pivotal to an understanding of dependency among older people. But, it is argued, it was between the 1920s and the 1960s that a major reconstruction of old age began to take place (Cole, 1992). It was predicated on the assumption that most old people could not contribute significantly to the 'real world'; that is, to the labour market. It is perhaps not surprising, therefore, that in the present social order, in which considerable value is placed upon individual responsibility, dependency is bound to be experienced as failure; or, as Leonard put it: 'being a nuisance, including becoming incontinent, often produces guilt and blame in the old person' (Leonard, 1975, p. 191).

Thus social constructions of old age are in part determined by the concept of 'usefulness to society'. Developing this theme, Peck stated:

Seventy years was an appropriate term of probation for man; longer life spans would benefit neither the individual nor the nation. It is an advantage to the world that men should die; that, having accomplished the great purpose of life, they should give place to others. (Peck, 1981, p. 5).

As a result of cultural transmission, the construction placed by society on death and dying in turn affects people's experience of the end of life. Thus,

The person who can look back on his life with satisfaction, knowing that on the whole he has done well, does not feel so strongly that he needs more time in which to develop unfulfilled potential, or to make amends . . . For him, death is not so threatening. He sees it more as a natural event, to mark the completion of his life. (Stedeford, 1984, p. 75).

Social constructions of death and dying also are inter-laced with prevailing cultural perspectives on life and living. This concept is reflected by Butler (1963):

. . . what we fear most is not really death but a meaningless and absurd life. I believe most human beings can accept the basic fairness of each generation's taking its turn on the face of the planet if they are not cheated out of the full measure of their own turn. The tragedy of old age in America is that we have made absurdity all but inevitable, we have cheated ourselves. (Butler, 1963, p. 422).

Others argue that society's quest for youth may be at the expense of deriving intrinsic pleasures from what some call the more spiritual wisdom of ageing. As a result, the old become more concerned with disguising their age:

17

To remain active members of society and continue to do our share of life's work is a matter of vital concern to those of us who are classed as elderly people. (Smith, 1905, p. 1-2).

But a consistent theme in the literature is that, for most old people, the final stage of life is full of pain, isolation and diminished faculties.

Acceptance of death as 'the final stage'

For contemporary men and women it is difficult to see life in any other way than in stages, but for the fifteenth century citizen, for example, no meaning would have been attached to the relatively modern developmental period of, for example, 'adolescence'. It has been argued that only a small step was required to change the language from 'ages' to 'stages' of life and that this 'staging' metaphor was:

> . . . represented by the emergent iconographic shape of the life cycle, where each step became a stage for the performance of certain roles. (Cole, 1992, p. 24).

Ultimately, it seems, our acceptance of death is not determined simply by the process of physical decline. An argument reappearing in the literature is that, provided the allotted time is up, death - both our own and other peoples' - is 'accepted' (Cole, 1992). But by assuming that *older* people have an automatic acceptance of death commentators could be accused of over-simplifying the matter. For example, it is claimed by some (for example, Pardi, 1977) that those working with elderly people may know instinctively, or are actively made aware by individuals who are dying, of their readiness or acceptance of death:

> Most people . . . will appreciate the feeling that the elderly, as a general rule, need little counselling about death. Most elderly people then do not see death as something which will cheat them. Moreover, since they have always associated death and old age, they have a more or less resigned acceptance of its eventuality. (Pardi, 1977, p. 130).

One possible flaw in this argument is that it fails to acknowledge the value for some individuals of the need to reflect on their life, in order for the process of acceptance to begin: the old, as well as the young, may need to validate their lives prior to death. Brearley (1981) echoes the idea that, because older people see those around them die, they are better prepared than younger people and

18

thus should be less distressed. Whilst there is some evidence to support the notion that older people close to death are more likely to 'accept' death - 'as many as two thirds of those who died under fifty years of age were clearly apprehensive, whereas less than a third of those over sixty years were as anxious' (Hinton, 1972, p. 85) - it would be unwise to assume, just because someone is ninety years of age, for example, and 'accepts' the inevitability of his or her own death, that they are not terrified of *dying* or that they have no need to express and explore their thoughts, feelings and experiences. This tendency to assume that people accept death when older may mask other needs; and, it may further indicate 'death denied' (see Ariès, 1981).

Although Butler and Lewis (1981) conclude that old age is a time of reflection and reminiscence which 'coupled with a psychological disengagement . . . can diminish such losses as attachment to the things of the world', they stress also that it can be a time of dichotomised experiences . . . 'the sins of omission and commission for which an individual blames himself weigh heavy in the light of approaching death' (Butler and Lewis, 1981, p. 37). Whilst they argued for the existence of a naturally recurring process - what they termed the 'life review' - older people dying in residential care are only likely to talk about their past, provided such 'reminiscence work' is undertaken with skill and patience.

A time to die: . . . social or physical departure?

Just before the turn of the century Fowler went so far as to say that the 'gradual death of old age can be pleasurable', claiming that it is only *premature* death which is distressing (Fowler, 1850, p. 59).

The idea that death in old age is experienced differently from untimely death may in part be due to a process of disengagement with the world, such as the loss of friends, spouse, independence and mobility (Kearl, 1989). It has been argued that the 'predominant theory of social gerontology remains disengagement theory, which depicts the mutual parting of the ways between society and its older members' (Cumming and Henry, 1961, p. 125). But it is possible also to argue that the institutionalisation of the death process *encourages* disengagement, the residential home thus becoming a secret place for the old to die (Kearl, 1989).

In recognising the incrementalism of the death process, Ariès concluded that 'death has ceased to be a moment' (Ariès, 1974, p. 53). Thus, there is a link between 'social' and 'physical' death (Prior, 1989). Bromley (1966) had suggested already that, in ideal circumstances, the process of decline should be graded to suit the declining biological and psychological capacities of the

19

individual on the one hand, and the needs of society on the other. Normal disengagement seems to lessen the fear of death (Bromley, 1966).

There has been a long history of the preparation for and expectations of old age. Calvanist ministers, for example, stressed the 'physical infirmities and social loss of age' (Cole, 1992, p. 140). The theme of a 'ripeness' for death was developed by Capon (1956) by reflecting a view mentioned earlier: that there is also a broader societal acceptance, or even expectation, of when death should ideally occur.

'Social' death is also equated with 'physical' death by other authors. Butler, for example, stated that 'sociability is seen to reside in human consciousness and the absence of such consciousness is regarded as being equivalent to death' (Butler, 1969, p. 157). It is perhaps this social death, more so than physical decline, which, for some people, ultimately makes death seem welcome (Pardi, 1977); but perhaps its acceptance adds weight to the view sometimes offered that death comes as 'a blessed relief'. In addition, for older people dying in institutional care the isolation may be compounded: 'For elderly individuals, already segregated from society . . . loneliness is most likely to be experienced as a problem', and this 'can be partially attributed to the social value placed on the dying old' (Kearl, 1989, p. 487). It may be that, as a result of this 'acceptance', 'their quiet exit scarcely raises a ripple on the sea of life' (Porter, 1842, quoted in Dickenson and Johnson, 1993).

During the 1970s a consensus emerged among health and social professionals - as well as among some researchers - who proposed the view that old people are (or should be) 'healthy', 'sexually active', 'engaged', 'productive', and 'self-reliant' (Fries and Crapo, 1981; Comfort, 1977; Tenenbaum, 1979). Although possibly founded on a desire to counter ageist attitudes this viewpoint has, inadvertently perhaps, fed the Victorian principle of a 'good' old age being dependent upon a person having lived a virtuous life. In attempting to counter ageism, the 'optimists' are in danger of perpetuating the quest for youth - or at least for a 'perpetual middle age',

> Since roughly the 1920's . . . existentially vital images of the ages and the journey of life, the middle-class American vision of ageing has amounted to a kind of perpetual middle age, at once valued above and disconnected from childhood and old age. (Maxwell, 1968, pp. 381).

Maxwell argues that the need for this 'vision' offers further evidence of implied ageism, as a result of the denial of old age, and suggests a broad cultural denial of death. It pays little cognisance, the author continues, to the positive aspects to old age, and merely reiterates society's value for youth and vigour.

After examining various studies Finley (1982) argued that a dispute was apparent among researchers about the treatment of elderly people by society and that distinctions have not always been made between professed attitudes toward old people, their status in society and their actual treatment. Old age in residential care is a time of emotional and physical dependence, when older people 'lean in trembling feebleness upon staff, to sink into the helplessness of second childhood' (Cole, 1992, p. 230) but many writers appear to ignore the implications of such features.

3 Dying in residential care

Monuments to age

The history of institutional care can be traced back to the early Christians, following the commandment of mercy and compassion (Townsend, 1964), but it was not until 1601 that Poor Houses were established under the Poor Relief Act. The philosophy was harsh because, 'if the staff had been kindly and sympathetic rather than repressive, and if the food . . . had been better, more people would have applied for admission (Townsend, 1964, p. 14). To reverse this, in 1947 Aneurin Bevan declared 'we have decided to make a great departure in the treatment of old people. The workhouse is to go'. Along with this courageous statement Bevan suggested that homes should be restricted to 25 or 30 people (Townsend, 1964). He added that it was not enough merely to reduce the number of residents; it was also necessary to change the relationship between the carers and the 'cared for'. 'The old "master and inmate" relationship is being replaced by one more nearly approaching that of an hotel manager and his guests' (Townsend, 1964, p. 19).

Thomson (1991) suggests that the workhouse was not a major source of *care* for older people - merely their place of residence - citing them as unpleasant places which were 'highly significant in dragooning the poor' (Thomson, 1991, p 207).

As a result of more middle-class older people being made homeless after the second world war, because their homes had been bombed, residential care needed improvements (Townsend, 1964). An enduring principle today is that homes should be 'small, homelike, and represent no loss of liberty' (Rackstraw, 1944). However, after the war it was also envisaged that places should be available on demand. There was no suggestion that homes should be restricted to very frail older people who lacked family or community support (National Assistance Bill, 1948 - Second reading).

Stern's observations of such places, deemed to be 'homes' for older people, are somewhat cynical:

> Unlike some primitive tribes, we do not kill off our aged and infirm. We bury them alive in institutions. To save our faces, we call the institutions homes - a travesty on the word. I have seen dozens of such homes in the last six months - desolate places peopled with blank-faced men and women, one home so like the other that each visit seemed a recurrent nightmare. (Stern, 1947, p. 17).

Victor's more recent findings do little to stimulate confidence that the situation has changed a great deal: 'there is little contact with the wider community. Domestic activities are also restricted, with residents generally given very little control over most aspects of their lives' (Victor, 1987).

Summarising Goffman's work, Jones and Fowles (1984) remind us that anyone who cannot,

> vote with their feet, for reasons of sickness, infirmity, age, fear of the consequences or lack of a viable alternative, cannot leave. In that sense, long-stay patients in general hospitals or residents in old people's homes may be as surely institutionalised as those confined by lock and key. (Jones and Fowles, 1984, p. 201).

Baldwin and her colleagues, however, are strongly critical of the concept of institutionalisation when applied indiscriminately; they are critical particularly of the 'induced dependency hypothesis', which argues that 'the more institutional regimes deny residents' control over their lives, the more they tend to foster their dependency' (Booth, 1985, p. 3 cited in Baldwin et al, 1993, p. 72). Their criticism are threefold. Firstly,

> . . . it is no longer helpful to assume that there is one institutionalisation process which in all essential respects is little affected by culture, the economic context, the service orientation in which a residential establishment is located and so on. (p. 74).

Secondly, the existence of residents as a captive audience is too convenient for researchers wedded to an explanation of events based on 'institutionalisation', for one reason because,

> . . . many situations in which people depend on others for their care are far removed from the idealised myths about supportive family life. Interactive

processes may be at work in such situations which may be comparable to those typically regarded as only existing in institutions. (p. 75).

And thirdly,

> The structured dependency thesis, which emerged out of the political economy of ageing, has been widely regarded as one of the most important contributions to social gerontology because it located dependency in the context of the wider inequalities experienced by older people, inequalities which are carried over from earlier in the lifecycle. (pp. 75-76).

Baldwin et al (1993) acknowledge that both Booth (1985) and Willcocks et al (1987) draw upon the notion of 'structured dependency', but only in a limited way and only in respect of 'post-admission effects'. However, for Baldwin and her colleagues 'structured dependency is a concept which has the capacity to broaden out the study of institutionalisation' (p. 76) although they believe that it has limitations 'because of its lack of attention to human agency' (p. 76). Rejecting the notion of applying universally the institutionalisation hypothesis to *all* institutions, they conclude that,

> A more productive way forward may be found in moving away from the concept of institutionalisation and focusing instead on the degree of dependency (and independence and interdependence) which exists for older people in any care situation; formal or informal, residential or community-based.' (p. 77).

Finally, they quote Phillipson (1986) as having provided a link between the study of institutionalisation and other issues which are pivotal to the whole field of gerontology when he proposed,

> . . . the need to develop a gerontology which successfully links biography with class structure, personality and social change and physical and mental ageing with cultural norms and attitudes. (Phillipson, 1986, p. 96).

In this context, their argument is that as a result of their different membership of various social and cultural groups different people experience care processes and environments *differently*: 'Institutionalisation: Why blame the institution?' they ask.

The effects of the community care legislation

It is important to consider briefly the effects of recent changes in social policy designed to reduce the number of people needing to enter residential care as a result of the Conservative government's 'Care in the Community' initiative and following the implementation of the National Health Service and Community Care Act, 1990. In respect of social work these effects are given a comprehensive overview in a recent work by Payne (1995).

Longman (1987) suggests that there is a crisis in the welfare state which reflects on residential care generally and, more specifically, upon its future direction for older people. The author suggests that institutionalisation reinforces the de-socialisation of older people while still salving the conscience of younger people. A further, relevant point is made that with the inception of 'community care' older people may be institutionalised and isolated within their own homes, becoming totally dependant on pre-determined services and thus reinforcing social isolation and the likelihood of disengagement (Longman, 1987). Although there were (and arguably still are) problems associated with residential care, the alternative is no less problematic:

> By default, the influential institutionalisation studies of the 1980s lend weight to an uncritical view of the superiority of care in the community which may not be borne out in reality. (Baldwin et al, 1993, p. 75).

Referring to Western culture, Dinnage concludes chillingly that 'never before have people died as noiselessly and hygienically as today in (these) societies, and never in social conditions so much fostering solitude' (Dinnage, 1990).

Furthermore, feminist writers such as Finch and Groves (1983) and Qureshi and Walker (1989) have highlighted some of the problematic features of community care, which include the over-representation of women amongst carer groups - including residential staff.

Residential care for older people and dependency levels

With the arrival of the new health and welfare services in 1948 less rigid distinctions between the two became apparent (Bloch and Parry, 1982). This led to a blurring of what constitutes hospital care and residential care. Hinton (1972) suggested that this lack of clarity affects how illness is defined,

> most people who do not die at home, end their lives in hospitals or institutions for the chronic sick. In fact, those to be considered as

'chronically sick' euphemistically include people with fatal cancers and other conditions. (Hinton, 1972, p. 36).

Summarising Burritt et al (1983), Victor (1987) considers the question of which institution cares for the chronically sick, and recognises the dilemma residential homes have in caring for very dependant residents, which centres upon the extent to which they can provide nursing care:

> Levels of disability in all types of residential care are high and estimates indicate that up to a quarter of those in residential care would be better cared for in hospital. (Victor, 1987).

Many writers confirm a rise in dependency levels in residential care (Kearl, 1989; Victor, 1987; Willcock et al, 1982; and Burritt et al, 1983). Also the age of residents on admission is rising in the Homes studied; and national figures in 1986 suggested that it was 85.1 years for women and 83.2 years for men (Phillipson and Walker, 1986).

As we saw in the Introduction the issue of dependency is seen as ambiguous by Booth et al (1983b), who questioned whether there had been a change in the proportion of residents who were substantially disabled. They acknowledged, however, that there was an increase in the proportion of residents classed as 'moderately dependant' and went on to suggest that the perceived increase in dependency within homes was 'probably due to an increase in the number of residents with intermediate needs for care'. They also suggested that, whilst there is a group which improves with care, it is balanced by a group who do not and that this situation works to produce 'broadly the same pattern of dependency from one year to the next' (Booth et al, 1983b, p. 219). Booth and his colleagues highlighted the implications of these findings for staffing levels. However, as Glaser and Strauss (1965a) found, inhibiting factors exist which lead to less than ideal circumstances. They result from 'institutional necessities, resources and the prevailing organisation of treatment - in the ideologies that can be tolerated or implemented within an institution' (Glaser and Strauss, 1965a). Amplifying this point, Hinton found that,

> poorer homes for the aged, can provide a half-concealed, ill-tended shuffle from life. Sick and elderly people are often admitted to poorly staffed, poorly designed . . . homes at a time when the care they need can just about be managed. (Hinton, 1972).

Other studies suggest that, as perceived by staff, the concept of resident dependency may be confusing. They conclude that the institution itself may

26

'create' dependency and thus the actual level of deterioration may have been exaggerated (Willcocks et al, 1982; Wade et al, 1983). Nevertheless, longitudinal studies have produced some evidence to confirm that admissions were for a markedly less fit group (Charlesworth and Wilkin, 1982). Potentially, the implications are at least twofold: firstly, a rise in both the number and rate of deaths might be expected and, secondly, that the ratio between medium and high dependency in each Home will play a big part in determining the actual number of deaths (Meacher, 1974; Booth, 1985). Booth explored the possibility that the regime within individual homes might have an effect on mortality and found that 'death rates in homes and the influence of homes with "positive" regimes as opposed to "institutionally-oriented" regimes seems low (or inconclusive)' (Booth, 1985). These studies also illustrate how dependency within Homes appears to change over time, thus the conclusions drawn by Booth and his colleagues in 1983 may need to be updated.

Other authors believe that the perceived rise in dependency and the consequent rise in the number of deaths has an effect on staff. They acknowledge that there is a need for 'a high standard of personal integrity and morale among a staff adequate in numbers and equipped with enough material facilities, if they are not to degenerate into awful places' (Hinton, 1972, p. 157), but Kearl went so far as to say that the trend is to recruit people who are 'employed off the street' . . . and are . . . 'at the bottom of the health care ladder' (Kearl, 1989). Staff appreciate that residents are older and frailer when admitted to residential care and are conscious that they often feel ill-equipped to offer the care that ideally they would prefer to provide (Willcocks et al, 1982). And when demands on staff time are, in reality, task-oriented, little space remains for the social and spiritual needs of residents (Power et al, 1983).

Responding to older people in residential care who are dying

Key implications emerge from Sudnow's ethnographic studies of death and dying in two hospitals in the United States when applied to residential care for older people. He noticed for example that much effort was spent in keeping alive those deemed to be 'special cases' although far less time was spent with the 'socially unworthy' (Sudnow, 1967). Similarly, Glaser and Strauss (1965a) earlier had found that dying patients were expected to meet two kinds of obligations: firstly, they should not attempt to bring about or hasten their own deaths and, secondly, they should behave in a courageous and 'decent' manner. It seems easier for staff working in institutions to appreciate those who die with courage and who do it gracefully, possibly because it leads to less emotional

27

stress but also it may enable those caring for the dying person to feel useful professionally. Vachon (1987) describes the positive and negative aspects of both involvement and attachment but identified *over*-involvement as a source of stress.

Hockey (1990) describes vividly the way elderly people in a residential home can be moved around when they become incontinent or unable to walk. The language used is stark and unsentimental when the author concluded that,

> (as they) become corpses, which is the unspoken end product of all social care homes, they were separated and placed in an alcove convenient for staff attention rather than joining the more able residents in the main lounges. (Bond and Bond, 1994, p. 177, referring to Hockey, 1990).

Bond and Bond (1994) continue as follows:

> Surprisingly James (1986) also observed people in a hospice attached to a hospital also moved into a single room as death approached. The distancing and separation of dying people in institutional care is a microcosm of the less obvious but powerfully pervasive death-distancing strategies in our society at large. (Bond and Bond, 1994, p. 177).

Glaser and Strauss (1965b) devised the term 'awareness contexts' to identify the extent to which people knew whether or not they were dying. Four awareness contexts emerged: *closed awareness*, in which everyone else but the patient knows; *suspicion awareness*, in which the patient suspects what others know; *mutual pretence awareness*, when everyone pretends others do not know; and finally, *open awareness*, in which knowledge of death and dying is shared. The point of their findings was to describe how the tactics used by professional staff with dying people altered depending upon which 'awareness context' applied.

Not surprisingly perhaps, the literature studied concludes that the way death and dying are handled is a function of the institution in which it occurs and in which the care is managed (and this appears to be the case even in the person's own home). Furthermore, central to the way dying residents are cared for is the extent to which they and their carers are aware of their location on the 'dying trajectory' (Glaser and Strauss, 1965b).

Another theme in the literature is that, as the dependency of residents increases, so too does their need for more specialised care when approaching the end of their life.

Residential care and the hospice movement

In the 1960s Cecily Saunders founded the British hospice movement, the philosophy of which is to recognise the uniqueness and importance of the dying person and their carers. The focus is on the 'person' rather than the 'illness', and the proponents of the modern hospice have attempted to redefine the word 'hospice' to signify a 'concept,' not a place (Littlewood, 1992). Put another way, it is a philosophy not a method of care. Specifically, this philosophy has been described as 'a way one may control one's life until death' (Kearl, 1989). The hospice was to be a safe place to think and grieve about death (Hinton, 1972). The finding that hospice patients seemed less anxious - and less depressed - than a comparable group of people dying in other institutions was, for some, not surprising (Hinton, 1972) given that in America in 1970, Kübler-Ross was promoting the need, and the right, of the dying person to talk openly about his or her feelings (Walter, 1992). However, although a proportion of hospice patients are older people, in one study of those cared for in hospices it was found that the majority of *patients* felt that the 'old are more compliant, amenable to institutional care, and possibly unable to benefit from hospice care' (Kearl, 1989). Thus, despite the ageism implied by such comments, if it were considered appropriate to transfer the concept of the hospice movement to residential care, this could prove difficult unless it was acknowledged openly that people entering Homes are in the last phase of their life. Although their condition is not usually deemed 'terminal', their needs appear to be similar to those who have been diagnosed as being 'terminally ill'.

. . . people's status as 'dying' is often only recognised when terminal illness is present. If it is not present, people are seen as 'living' even if seriously ill. If we are to raise the status of the care of the elderly in the same way the hospice movement has raised the status of cancer care, we may need to recognise that we are all at different stages on the road to death, with some nearer than others. (Walter, 1992, p. 53).

However, this idea is unlikely to be accepted readily by a society in which, as we have seen, many may prefer to deny death. Whilst the role of the hospice movement is broadly understood by society to be a place to which people 'go to die', residential homes are perceived overtly as places to 'go and live'. But an argument which appears regularly in the literature (see for example, Ariès, 1974) is that the social isolation created in such institutions places residents in the realms of the dead - at least to society at any rate. In fact, according to Kastenbaum and Aisenberg, rather than being provided with an appropriate environment and care, the terminally ill elderly person is more likely to be rejected as a deviant and denied control because being both old and dying is doubly stigmatising. (Kastenbaum and Aisenberg, 1972, p. 121).

Consequently staff confront daily the dilemma of caring for older people who are dying without public (and often medical) recognition of their terminal state.

The lack of congruence between the training of hospice workers and that of residential workers may affect significantly the quality of the final stages of life for older people in residential care. While 'many nursing homes are well run by devoted proprietors who have had much training and experience' (Hinton, 1972) this may not be so in the majority of local authority residential homes:

Local authority homes are trying to cope simultaneously with two conflicting tasks: on the one hand, to provide comprehensive personal and sometimes nursing care to physically and mentally infirm old people, and on the other hand to create an environment for living that safeguards the dignity and personal freedom of more independent residents. (Booth, 1985).

Unlike the culture of the hospice, there are no set institutional practices about talking about death in residential homes; on the contrary, it may be true that 'unless the (resident) initiates conversation about impending death, no staff member is required to talk about it with him' (Zarit, 1978).

Ultimately it is likely to be the culture of the residential home which is pivotal in influencing (positively or negatively) the reactions of staff (Foster, 1985). And when this happens both staff and residents alike are likely to conform to the cultural norm of the Home (Davies and Knapp, 1981). Yet it has been noted that there is sometimes an unspoken 'rule' which operates within the sub-culture of the Home and which determines what - and how much - is said about death and dying. Often it is influenced by the medical profession and this is why it has been termed 'the doctor-nurse game' (Stein et al, 1990, p. 547) - because it is played by doctors and nurses with patients. The 'game' is enacted within residential homes for older people in so far as their of *is* the care of the dying (Walter, 1992):

The practical implications of this are that people who currently consider themselves to be working with 'the elderly' are also working with 'the dying'. This can no longer be solely the province of those working with people medically predicted as having but a short time to live. (Walter, 1992, p. 293).

30

Hockey's study compared residents who were dying in old people's homes and in a hospice. Referring to Hockey's findings Bond and Bond noted that,

> there was much greater control over all aspects of life mediated through the asymmetrical distribution of power between staff and residents and a greater separation of life from death. In the independent hospice there was far less separation, more autonomy for patients with control related to symptoms, and . . . care offering unconditional support to patients and staff. (Bond and Bond, 1994, p. 186).

The routinisation of daily-living tasks in residential care

The daily events in a residential home can create a culture of silence regarding death and dying. Uniforms, routines, and other events such as bath times and meal times, as well as 'rooms just like home' support the 'enactment of normality' when things are far from 'normal' (De Beauvoir, 1972). Others also contend that the culture engendered by imposed routines can erode autonomy and affect the ability of residents to express their wishes (see Lidz and Fischer, 1992, for example). It has also been argued that this loss of autonomy may further reflect the way society disengages from older people and the dying (Kearl, 1989).

Kearl (1989) concludes that 'what we think of a person influences how we will perceive him; how we perceive him influences how we will behave toward him; and how we behave toward him ultimately influences who he becomes' (Kearl, 1989, p. 472). Although consumer studies of residential care encounter reliability problems, nevertheless Lerner found that four out of every five older people in institutional settings agreed that 'they are at the mercy of staff, compelled to conform to rules and regulations that may be contrary to their own needs and desires, dying socially while waiting for the end to come' (Lerner, 1970). It is this, in part, which Goffman concluded constituted his notion of the 'total institution' (Goffman, 1961):

> A basic social arrangement in modern society is that the individual tends to sleep, play, and work in different places with different co-participants, under different authorities, and without an over-all rational plan. The central features of total institutions can be described as a breakdown of the barriers ordinarily separating these three spheres of life. (Goffman, 1961, pp. 5-6).

Similarly, some argue that loss of control on entering an institution further

31

inhibits the ability to make known one's needs (Levine and Scotch, 1970). The ritual of the 'hair-do' and the 'making-up' of residents further reinforces the idea of society abandoning residents to 'immerse themselves within the socially prescribed activities which allow them to forget . . .' (Kearl, 1989). It has also been suggested that non-conformity would be to deny the 'institutional map and thus be seen as abnormal' (Wilson, 1939). De Beauvoir goes further, arguing that 'the audience must participate, if only symbolically', and that 'mutual pretence is done with terrible seriousness, for the stakes are very high' (De Beauvoir, 1972, p. 271). Somewhat frighteningly, residents absorb the culture of the Home quickly.

On entering residential care there is a covert understanding that an elderly person will end their days there, and yet often it is not considered 'decent' to broach the subject of how they wish to be cared for when dying, and what services the Home offers (Hinton, 1972; Townsend, 1964). Hinton (1972) observed further that there was a veil of silence in some residential homes. A game is thus devised, with its own unspoken rules and rituals. The masquerade which ensues is complicated; role expectations are high, and each 'actor makes the role easier to play' (Glaser and Strauss, 1965b, p. 273).

It appears that the decision whether or not to talk about death rests largely with staff but that 'it is the old who are most likely to think about and discuss death and who are least likely to be frightened by it' (Kearl, 1989 p. 467). But when replicating the work of Macdonald and Dunn (1982), Ashby et al (1991) found that, among people *wishing* to die, there was an *increased* risk of distress, of approximately the same magnitude as that for depression. Unfortunately it is not known whether this may have been as a result of existing depression and distress among such people which, wholly or partly, led them to want to die in the first place.

In a similar vein, a body of research into the verbal behaviour of nurses in communication with cancer patients has shown that the majority block direct questions concerning death and dying and ignore patients' cues to take the conversation into what are seen as painful areas (Field, 1989; Wilkinson, 1991). Thus part of the reason for maintaining the masquerade is to protect all of the players: the resident, staff members and the family. For residents, the pretence allows them to act as if they were not dying; for staff and for the family it helps reduce the fear of the resident 'going to pieces' (Glaser and Strauss, 1965a). When residents openly express a willingness to die, a tension is created because 'staff members persistently insist on the pretence that the patients are going to recover' (De Beauvoir, 1972, p. 276).

Durkheim (1968) focused on the integration of individuals into communal life and argued that beliefs and ideas play a significant role. Collectively-held beliefs imposed culturally on macro-society, and on the micro-society of the residential

32

home, ultimately, it is argued, create the barriers which prevent communication, even though it is widely acknowledged that people 'gain great relief from unburdening themselves of fears, grief, feelings of guilt and failure, of loneliness or of frustration at being dependant on others' (Elias, 1985). Sharing such feelings can be consoling for residents, though rather uncomfortable for the listener; to render this service 'we have to be prepared to be disturbed' (Lamberton, 1980). In institutions where relationships are described as 'slender' (see Townsend, 1964) and when free choice is restricted significantly (see Faden and Beauchamp, 1986) then the likelihood of this being achieved appears slim. In such a culture it is possible that residents will choose to deny a closeness with staff; if power and independence are eroded residents then may retreat into the private world of the mind thereby retaining the last vestiges of control (De Beauvoir, 1972). They will have observed how death is dealt with in the Home (perhaps noting a lack of respect by staff who stand over residents, talking about them to others in his or her presence); consequently, they may feel patronised by being told 'not to worry' if they ask about a resident whom they know has died (Downie and Calman, 1987). Townsend, too, noted that what residents have observed about how death is treated will indicate to them how *they* may expect to be treated: 'they saw that their own death was likely to be equally undignified and anonymous' (Townsend, 1964).

The effect of death and dying among residents upon their carers

Questions exist concerning what happens to people who may be faced with one death after another (Stedeford, 1984). As Freud (1917 in Strachey, 1957) noted, it is likely that the more deaths experienced by people, the greater the need for the deployment of defence mechanisms - in particular adaptation. It is possible that frequent losses blunt the expression (and perhaps ultimately the feeling) of grief: 'the saturation with sorrow and the bitter necessity to adapt and carry on, reduce the intensity of grief over repeated tragedies' (Hinton, 1972, p. 174). This phenomenon is mirrored by Stedeford (1984) who argued, like Saunders (1965) earlier, that many are drawn to the work, and that certain motives (such as compassion) may help them overcome 'that part of their nature that would naturally turn away' (Stedeford, 1984, p. 166).

It has been acknowledged that those who work in residential care with older people tend to be those with few (if any) qualifications (Twining, 1988). There are concerns about whether they are equipped to deal effectively with dying people. It is suggested that education in the caring professions has tended to neglect this area of care (Brearley, 1981). However, Poss (1981) warns that dealing with this difficult task is more complex than perhaps can be covered by education alone:

> The accumulation of mere facts regarding dying and terminal care is unlikely to constitute adequate training for the task. (Poss, 1981, p. 44).

Greenwood (1966) and Harrington (1977) introduced the notion that the 'professionalisation' (see, for example, Larson, 1977) of those dealing with death simply reaffirms society's fears about death thereby reinforcing its unnaturalness:

> The more sophisticated we become, the more unnatural death becomes and the more ingenious become our rationalizations to explain it away. (Harrington, 1977, p. 194).

There has been some debate in the literature about the extent to which death and dying leads to the suppression of feelings among staff. Some people may be equipped more naturally to deal with the task; they may have an aptitude for speaking easily and honestly to people who are dying. However, the culture of the residential or institutional setting can quickly inhibit this ability (Glaser and Strauss, 1965b). As previously discussed, the culture of the institution exerts many influences, both at a macro-societal level in relation to attitudes to older people - and specifically to death and dying - and at a micro-level within the institution itself. However, it is acknowledged that even though staff may become accustomed to death it is not always the case that people inevitably become 'hardened' to it: 'in a sense they become used to death, not hardened, but able to cope with more prolonged exposure to it' (Stedeford, 1984, p. 166).

But it is considered by some authors that staff are not merely *adapting* to very painful situations. A complex range of forces are present including: the culture and the personality of the carer; their own life experiences and belief systems; whether staff feel 'impersonalised' behind a uniform (see Martin, 1989); and personal defence mechanisms which are used to divert painful feelings of loss and grief. In the early 1960s a number of authors argued that avoidance of the acknowledgement of death within residential care can result from unresolved feelings of grief (Birley, 1960) and little has emerged to contradict this. Such 'denial' is seen ultimately as being to the detriment of the dying person. Continuing in the psychodynamic spirit of the earlier writers, Hinton argues that,

> He may be surrounded by people whose every manifest word or action is

designed to deny or avoid the fact that he is dying, and he is aware of the artificiality of their deception. (Hinton, 1972, p. 127).

It is further posited that, not only is this denial detrimental to the dying person, it also has the potential to affect the well-being of the staff member. And, in describing the failure to talk about death as the 'conspiracy of silence', Thompson concludes that it affects 'subsequent bereavement and its management' (Thompson, 1993).

A balance between having sufficient insight and sensitivity by staff into their own and the resident's feelings is considered necessary by many authors. Similarly the need for appropriate defence mechanisms to cope with the prospect of working with dying residents is also thought to be important by some authors (for example, Brearley, 1981). Confusingly, although denying or suppressing one's emotions is thought to be damaging, both psychologically and sociologically (Kearl, 1989), Walter (1992) suggests that perhaps denial is the 'only alternative' if staff are not to experience too much pain.

Stedeford (1984) concluded that to care for dying people properly staff must face their own mortality: 'we care for dying patients best when we have allowed ourselves to contemplate our own mortality, and do not have to shy away from theirs'. This view supports Poss's assertion that 'while workers are afraid of death they are likely to convey this to patients' (Poss, 1981, p. 48).

The relationship which the carer has with the resident prior to death influences feelings of loss. The length of time the worker has known the resident and the nature of the care given may also be significant (Stedeford, 1984). She goes on to describe the dangers of suppressing grief, which ultimately affects health and well-being. The suppression of grief within the culture of a residential home can set the tone for the group, which may then influence how individuals behave within it. Anyone breaking the 'rules' may engender misunderstanding or even hostility (Gorer, 1965). Hinton (1972) further proposed that grief can become displaced if its free expression is not permitted, and that excessive grief may emerge when a second (perhaps lesser) bereavement period begins (see, for example, Murray-Parkes, 1972; 1988). Gorer (1965) developed further this process of avoidance, and argued that many staff adopt a 'stiff upper lip' when experiencing bereavement. For example, 'mourners' may not be allowed to be thoughtful or sad if their colleagues constantly pressurise them to come 'out of themselves':

Giving way to grief is stigmatized as morbid, unhealthy, demoralizing - very much the same terms are used to reprobate mourning as were used to reprobate sex; and the proper action of a friend and well-wisher is felt to be the distraction of a mourner from his or her grief . . . (Gorer, 1965, p. 113).

Although Gorer seems to have been the first to posit the idea that it is the lack of ritual connected with death which contributes to the public repression of grief and mourning (Gorer, 1965), Elias suggested that the way grief is expressed is founded on the idea of a male preserve, and that this now needs updating. He argues that contemporary society distrusts ritual and formality, so these are no longer available as ways of expressing grief. He goes on to suggest that it is the 'Anglo-Saxon male form of modernity' which fosters 'a certain reserve, so many of us are unwilling to express ourselves personally either' (Elias, 1985, p. 36).

The implications of the above are significant, and complex: to care for living and dying elderly people in a sensitive way, so as to recognise their many needs at the last phase of life, may involve dismantling the myriad cultural and personal barriers bounded by cultural norms and expectations. Unfortunately too, what little research exists in this field is equally pessimistic. For example a recent study by the Royal College of Nursing (1992) warned that people in residential homes were being denied skilled nursing care when they were dying. On the whole, the literature offers little room for optimism:

> Increasingly, the quality of life during the year before death is going to depend on the attributes of residential homes and their staff. (Cartwright, 1991).

Part Two
RESEARCH FINDINGS

'Not to lament, not to curse, but to understand'.

Spinoza

4 Methodology

Methodological discussion and implications

Broadly speaking two methodological schools exist, between, on the one hand, *quantitative* approaches, which seek to test correlations between variables, and, on the other, *qualitative* approaches, which are concerned more with observation, description and exploration (see Silverman, 1993). Silverman concludes, however, that 'unfortunately the two schools have sometimes been defined as polar opposites' (p. 22). This tendency to polarise quantitative and qualitative methods of social enquiry is also regretted by Hammersley (1993): 'while we must recognise that there are some profound differences in approach, it is important to keep methodological discussions open' (p. xiii).

In the present study, however, qualitative methodology was selected for much the same reason as Van Maanen (1979) articulated: 'to uncover and explicate the ways in which people in particular work settings come to understand, account for, take action and otherwise manage their day-to-day situation' (quoted in Miles and Huberman, 1994, p. 8). Thus, because the aim was to understand and explore the ways in which carers in residential homes *made sense of their experiences* when caring for older people in the later stages of life, a qualitative research methodology was chosen. Additionally, the selection of qualitative methodology was adopted as a result of the paucity of research in this area. In doing so, however, Silverman's concern was acknowledged: he is critical of those (and cites Singleton et al, 1988, as an example) who see qualitative methodology only as 'a relatively minor methodology to be used, if at all, at early or exploratory stages of a study '(p. 20). This concern over the marginalisation of qualitative methodology was also echoed by Sankar and Gubrium (1994) when applying it to the field of ageing research: 'Qualitative research is a distinct orientation, with its own analytic traditions and methodologies, and it cannot be reduced to or understood as a precursor to quantification' (p. x).

Most writers on research methodology conclude that defining qualitative research has proved difficult. They prefer instead to identify 'defining characteristics' rather than attempt an all-encompassing and exhaustive definition (see Silverman, 1993). Miles and Huberman (1994, p. 10) outline such characteristics as: (i) a focus on 'naturally occurring, ordinary events in natural settings' in order to produce what they called 'a strong handle on what *real life* is like'; (ii) a confidence 'buttressed by local groundedness', that is, 'the fact that the data are collected in close proximity to a specific situation, rather than throughout the mail or over the phone' (thus, and somewhat confusingly, Miles and Huberman employ a slightly different meaning for 'grounded' than that originally used in 1967 by Glaser and Strauss); (iii) offering 'richness and holism'; and (iv) that such data are well-suited for 'locating the meanings people place on events, processes, and structures of their lives . . . and for connecting these meanings to the social world around them'. Again, it was this last characteristic which was of particular importance to the nature of the enquiry best suited to this study.

The central aim of the research

Before moving on to consider how the data were collected and analysed it is important to crystallise the central aim of the study. The key question which the research sought to understand was *'What are the experiences of a small number of carers for older people in residential homes during the later stages of life?'*

The aim of this qualitative research study, therefore, was to explore those experiences and analyse them thematically.

Data collection: selecting the interviewees

Following a verbal and written explanation to the senior manager with overall responsibility for residential care, the Officer-in-Charge in each of nine Homes within one local authority social services department was contacted by telephone. Eventually, five Homes agreed to take part. The Officers-in-Charge were asked to give an open invitation to staff (to include themselves and the officer team) in which staff were asked to indicate if they were willing to be interviewed. After two weeks a second telephone call was made to each Home in order to identify those who were interested in participating. Another letter was sent giving details of the research. Appointments were then made for the interviews to take place. Asking officers in charge to select those staff who appeared most articulate or vocal was considered. However, this approach would have excluded a valuable source of information, and could have been seen to value only those who are used to expressing themselves. Ultimately I felt that it was my task, as the interviewer, to help respondents express what they thought and felt rather than to set out deliberately to be selective.

Confidentiality and the right of privacy were considered carefully, especially as interviewees were asked to explore and discuss their views and feelings on this sensitive subject.

When selecting interviewees consideration was given to the question of whether to include them if they had experienced a recent personal bereavement. However, it was considered important to interview all who volunteered and then to deal with any distress at the time.

Another methodological difficulty was encountered when deciding whether to interview staff while they were on duty. The nature of the topic could lead to distress, and might cause heightened emotional states which possibly would make returning to work difficult. In an earlier study in 1990 Cartwright and Seale faced this methodological problem and stated,

> Most worrying from an ethical point of view were the occasional situations where an interview proceeded without much emotional arousal, but the emotional impact was felt afterwards by the respondent. (Cartwright and Seale, 1990, p. 55).

On the other hand, it would have been difficult to interview staff in their own time because there was no facility to pay them. This in turn would have been likely to affect their willingness to participate, and thus limit the number of respondents.

Although it was possible that, if they viewed it merely as a welcome break in their routine, staff might agree to be interviewed while at work, in view of the nature of the topic it was felt unlikely that anyone would volunteer for this reason. Indeed, the depth of feeling expressed by staff suggested that those who volunteered felt they had 'something to say', and seemed very willing to participate. It is difficult to say whether those who did not volunteer lacked interest in being interviewed; they may simply not have been ready or willing to talk about their experiences.

Consideration was given to interviewing other people involved within their work with death and dying - for example, nurses, hospice workers, doctors or priests. This idea was rejected, however, because it was not an aim of the research to conduct a comparative study.

In deciding how the data should be collected consideration was given to

41

asking interested staff to keep a diary of feelings and experiences prior to being interviewed. This was rejected, however, for two reasons: firstly, some staff might not feel confident or competent to do so; secondly, they would have had to spend time compiling it at work (which was considered impractical). Another way of eliciting the experiences of staff would have been to interview them during the last few hours before a resident died and then immediately after a resident's death. In addition to the obvious problem of predicting when a resident might die - not to mention the ethical questions of asking staff to be interviewed when they should have been concentrating solely upon the resident - also it would have been difficult logistically to interview people directly following the death of a resident because of the time pressures involved in conducting the research on a part-time basis. On reflection, as the research did not seek to find out the reaction of staff at the point of a resident's death - rather, it was concerned to explore the overall experience of caring for people who die, in the context of their relationship with that resident and their own life experiences - then this approach to data collection was rejected. Naturally, participant observation was not considered appropriate due to the intimate nature of residential care generally, and in respect of care to people who are dying in particular, and because of significant ethical and moral dilemmas surrounding this area of research. Finally, the idea of group interviews was also discarded because individuals were thought likely to respond differently in front of colleagues, partly as a reflection of group norms and cultures within specific Homes and partly as a function of the powerful nature of the subject of death and dying.

The interviews, therefore, were planned by prior appointment on an individual basis in the residential home in which the staff member worked. All those who were on duty were given the time by their manager to be away from their work duties. Two members of staff said they preferred to be interviewed in their own time. Whilst most interviewees had appointments, three presented themselves for interview when I was in the Home interviewing other staff. Everyone who took part in the research was interviewed in the Home where they worked in a room which offered privacy.

Data collection: interviewees' profile

A total of twenty staff members in five Homes formed the research group. Three interviewees were of officer grade with the remaining seventeen comprising care assistants on manual worker grade. Seventeen interviewees were female and three were male. All but one of the interviewees had left school at the age of sixteen or below and all had either had no paid employment prior to taking up their post - for example, they had been at home looking after the family, had been unemployed or made redundant - or they had been employed in other jobs which were said by the interviewee to have failed to produce sufficient job satisfaction.

The age range of the interviewees was twenty six to sixty years (the mean age being 44.7 years, with a standard deviation of 9.94 years). The length of service ranged from two to fifteen years (producing a mean length of service of 6.52 years, and a standard deviation of 3.98 years).

Data collection: conducting the interviews

A semi-structured interview schedule was designed in order to give interviewees ample scope to express their *own* thoughts and feelings while simultaneously providing a framework to cover different topics. The aim of the interview style, again partly as a consequence of the topic, was to establish a rapport. This style was considered by Oakley (1981) to be more likely to break down some of the barriers which might exist between two people, each of whom, as a direct consequence of their relative positions in an organisation, possesses or experiences formal authority and power differently. It was clear that eliciting responses from people who may have been unaccustomed to articulating feelings and ideas in a formalised way to others would require empathy and a level of 'positive regard' on my part; certainly I felt it was important for me to be encouraging. I claim no personal qualities which made it easy for them to talk to me, but I was both surprised and moved by their openness and honesty. It is not possible to say whether this was as a result of the experience of having an opportunity to talk, or a combination of other factors. Interestingly all of the women said they found it a good experience and thanked me for listening to them, but the men did not. However, care has been taken not to draw any conclusions from this; the question of gender difference is raised simply as an example of the myriad research possibilities surrounding the subject of providing care to people in the later stages of life.

The interviews were undertaken from April to July 1994, with the first two being conducted as pilot interviews in order to refine the themes and to identify any additional areas within the topic for future interviews. From the pilot interviews it was decided not to reject certain questions which, for those particular interviewees, did not produce detailed responses. This proved subsequently to have been an appropriate decision because other interviewees often said more in respect of these questions. It was decided also to include the two pilot interviews for analysis because each was considered to be appropriate within the context of the research methodology.

Each interview ranged in duration from one to two hours. Confidentiality was discussed before the interview began, and each interviewee was assured firstly of anonymity and secondly that there would be no feedback to anyone on his or her individual responses. Finally, they were reassured that the tapes would not be transcribed by anyone other than myself.

The interviews were recorded on audio-tape with the permission of the interviewee, and all were assured that if they did not want to keep the tape themselves when the research was complete then it would be erased by myself. Each interviewee was given my home and work telephone numbers and encouraged to contact me if they had anything they wanted to say or ask after the interview. Even though one interviewee did contact me following her interview, telling me that she had experienced some distress on returning home, many of the interviewees (including her) said they felt that they had benefited from talking about their feelings and experiences of looking after older people who die.

The possibility of opening up old wounds was very real in this research. Care was needed to achieve a balance between obtaining information which was relevant to the topic without inhibiting interviewees from expressing themselves fully. Sometimes it was necessary to explore individuals' experiences in their private lives which were relevant in order to see if and how they were related to their views about the older people for whom they cared, but even those interviewees who were affected emotionally during or following the interview said that they had enjoyed being interviewed. However, care was taken to make sure that interviewees were not exposed to distressing emotions which they would be left with after the interview. Consequently after the tape-recorder had been switched off they were debriefed in order to find out how they were feeling and to consider with them whether they felt able to resume their duties.

Data analysis

The overall approach to data analysis was to adopt Glaser and Strauss' (1967) concept of 'grounding' the data i.e. deliberately to relate them to the preoccupations, interests and concerns of the research subjects. Hence, in practice, the concept of grounding the data during the process of analysis gives a potency to the people who were interviewed. In this vein, even the term 'interviewee' is rejected by some qualitative researchers as denoting a passivity which they are at pains to overcome - it is noticeable, for example, that in his research on 'dying alone' Seale (1995) uses the term 'speakers', presumably because he believes that it empowers those who were interviewed far more than 'interviewee'. Miles and Huberman (1994) capture the essence of a 'grounded' approach in the following passage:

> From the start of data collection, the qualitative analyst is beginning to decide what things mean - is noting regularities, patterns, explanations, possible configurations, causal flows, and propositions. The competent researcher holds these conclusions lightly, maintaining openness and scepticism, but the conclusions are still there, inchoate and vague at first, then increasingly explicit and grounded, to use the classic term of Glaser and Strauss . . . (Miles and Huberman, 1994, p. 11).

Five of the six steps used by Miles and Huberman (1994) when analysing the data were applied to the transcripts. Summarised, the first four are:

1. Affixing codes to a set of field notes drawn from interviews;
2. Noting reflections or other remarks in the margins;
3. Sorting and sifting through these materials to identify similar phrases... patterns, themes and common sequences;
4. Elaborating a small set of generalisations that cover the consistencies discerned. (Miles and Huberman, 1994, p. 9).

The last of their steps - 'Confronting those generalisations with a formalised body of knowledge in the form of constructs or theories' (p. 9) - was treated in this research as an amalgamation of Parts One and Three. The fifth step - 'Isolating the patterns and processes, commonalities and differences, and taking them out to the field in the next wave of data collection' (p. 9) - was rejected because a second round of interviews was not considered feasible.

Transcripts of the tapes were made soon after each interview and the tapes listened to several more times before analysis began. Common themes were identified and colour-coded on each transcript. At first there emerged twelve distinct patterns from this analysis but they tended to accord more with what Miles and Huberman (1994) refer to as 'first order conceptions' i.e. conceptions which are 'more descriptive or factual in nature', an example of which (in respect to a study of criminal convictions) they give as the 'Number of arrests in a precinct'. Thus during the preliminary analysis of the tapes in the present study such 'first order' categories included for example, 'Need to say goodbye to the resident' or 'Need to be with the dying person and not leave them alone'.

Miles and Huberman (1994) go on to describe 'second order conceptions', an example of which they give as 'Positing the patrol officer's turf as a central idea'. Another way of capturing this is to use instead the example of 'apples',

45

'pears', 'cherries' etc. to constitute 'first-order' conceptions, with 'fruit' corresponding to the notion of a 'second-order' conception. Using this idea it was possible to distil three themes, which also incorporate the original twelve patterns. As a consequence of this process, over and above the specific content contained in the tapes, interviewees seemed to be speaking about their *attitudes*, their *feelings* or their *behaviour* in respect of providing care to older people dying in a residential home. These three themes constitute the remaining chapter titles in Part Two; most of the original twelve patterns are interwoven within each chapter as sub-headings. The general approach adopted has been to thematically analyse and describe the data in Part Two (leaving the discussion of the data to Part Three).

5 Attitudes to religious beliefs and their own ageing

Religious beliefs of staff in relation to death and dying

It was interesting to note that many interviewees, whilst initially professing to hold no religious beliefs, went on to say that they believed death was not the end and that they believed in a 'life after death'. Although some thought that religious belief could be a source of comfort for some residents - one interviewee observing that 'religion helps people (residents) not fear death' - for others it was nevertheless important that residents should retain the right *not* to be influenced by personal beliefs: 'I talk in general terms. If they haven't got your religious views it's not fair to push them on to other people'.

Because of the frailty and high dependency levels of residents, everyone interviewed believed that they were witnessing conditions in people which in the past were confined to staff in medical settings. For some interviewees, working with frail older people exposed questions about the purpose of life: 'I sometimes look at these people and think "Why are we here? - Earth is hell". I am angry with God'.

Because many older people in residential homes now remain there until death (rather than being transferred to hospital or a hospice) staff attend to the dying person in bed, turning them regularly, washing them and feeding them by spoon or through a pipette. During this, sometimes protracted, period of time the resident may become semi-conscious, become confused or distressed, suffer weight-loss, and possibly have an unpleasant odour as well. Staff caring for dying residents are guided by medical advice from the general practitioner who may visit occasionally, but with most medication being administered by residential staff. Other than for pain control, one care assistant viewed giving medication and feeding as prolonging life unnecessarily. Initially she questioned

47

the compassion of God but on reflection concluded, with some anger, that it was the medical profession who tested the endurance of the sufferer (and the carer) beyond that which she considered justifiable:

> I saw this person - and all it was, was a skeleton - and she was being fed with a dropper, and I thought, 'Gosh, they say there is a God, but it is some God who would allow this'. Then afterwards when I gave it some thought, I thought, 'even if there is a God, these people were meant to die long before now'. It is doctors; it is them who are advocating that they should be treated in bed every hour, and turned and fed - and she was just a skeleton, unconscious. Certainly if there is a God, it was certainly nothing to do with Him.

For another interviewee working in a residential home for older people provided a 'test of faith'. And she believed her faith helped her accept the death of residents,

> I do not react badly to death in the Home. My faith helps me. You do not realise how strong your faith is when it isn't put to the test - you have got your faith, but you don't know how strong it is until it comes down to the crunch. It's been a great comfort.

Also, she felt that her personal belief system gave her an optimistic attitude towards working with older people. Her experiences of dealing with death and dying had given her insights into suffering which, rather than dulling her optimism and compassion, had kindled it:

> Life is here to be experienced, good or bad. You can get something out of every experience, however bad it is. If you look at it in a positive way, you can get something good out of it.

She illustrated this 'optimistic' attitude when she described the recent death of a resident: 'Even though it was quite a disagreeable experience for him, it was also quite a rewarding one (for him)'.

A recurrent theme concerned the belief in the existence of an 'after-life', which appeared to provide some staff with a sense of comfort (although not everyone linked it with having religious beliefs). One said, 'I have got no religious views, but I do believe in life after death'. Another worker found solace in the notion that the degree to which the dead person was loved would ensure a reunion after death between him or her and the staff member: 'I believe there is another life, and if there's love between people we will meet up again somewhere - it is a great comfort.' The concept of reunion was taken a step further by one worker who, describing himself as a Spiritualist, said: 'When I've got a problem I talk to my (dead) uncle, and that's how I cope - some people would laugh'. He said that his belief that he can continue to communicate with the spirit of those he has known helps him come to terms with death. He went on to say 'I am a spiritual person, so coping with death is not a problem. I don't see death as the end - the spirit is just moving'.

Although religious belief - or at least a belief in a 'greater Being' or an after-life - brought comfort to some interviewees, for one there was a sense of sadness in her voice when she said that she could not believe in this. She said poignantly, 'I would like to believe in life after death, but once you've lived your life, what else is there?'

Some staff commented upon religious and cultural differences in the way death is dealt with in the Home, and in society generally. They tended to argue that the largely secular way of dealing with the dying and the dead, and the process of mourning, were unhelpful to them. One person recalled the support derived from the local Catholic community in Ireland when she was a child. She felt that English non-Catholics avoid talking about death, whereas in Ireland 'they have a celebration of the person's life'.

She associated an absence of religious belief with a culture which is 'embarrassed to talk about death, like they're frightened of something'. In a similar vein, a worker who was brought up as a child in the West Indies puzzled over the lack of religious ceremony which accompanies death in England, recalling the rituals she attended in the Caribbean where the family and friends of the dead person sat around for days, feasting and talking about them and apparently drawing comfort from doing so.

Views on their own ageing

Residents who were dying, were dying in old age. Therefore it was considered important to seek the views of residential workers about the ageing process as well as their thoughts on death and dying. The age range of interviewees was between 26 years and 60 years but it was apparent that their views on when they thought 'old age' began did not appear necessarily to be influenced by their own age.

Two divergent views emerged. The first group comprised those who specified the biblical 'three score years and ten' - a phrase which they used regularly - as constituting an appropriate life-span; the second group were those who did not view age as a chronological event but as a psychological and experiential process, and it is this group which is explored in more depth. One interviewee expressed this sentiment with the cliché 'You are as old as you feel' but those who perceived ageing to be a 'state of mind' tended to believe that becoming 'old' was largely something within a person's own control unless s/he was impeded by physical disability or mental illness. Keeping a 'young outlook' and maintaining interests were cited as ways of maintaining youth. If this was achieved then there was no reason to view people as 'old'. As one person said 'Old age is when you deteriorate - when you cannot see, walk, hear, and cannot cope on your own'. For one interviewee the realisation of her own increasing age became apparent only by seeing her reflection in the mirror. She said 'Sometimes I feel young inside, but when I look at myself I'm not'. This realisation had increased her ability to empathise with residents:

> Many times when we talk to the old, we talk about them - about what we are going to do with them, without explaining it to them. We should talk to them, but we don't - we talk over them, which is so easily done.

For some interviewees their own increasing age enabled them to feel that they understood the thoughts and fears of those they cared for in the Home. One said 'Sometimes I do understand how they feel as well because when you are getting older you feel more near to their state of mind, and so you can see how they feel'. She went on to say that getting old inevitably meant dying, and although she was grateful that she had escaped disease and death, she had retained her childhood fear of death:

> I've always been like that. I remember being . . . outside when I was a child and I used to sit and look at the stars, and death seemed so far away, and I was just afraid - I don't know why - I've just always been afraid.

Working with older people in a residential home often exposes staff to experiences which confront them with their own mortality. For one interviewee her fears of ageing had changed since she first went into 'care work'. Now she noticed a difference in her fears, which initially had been concerned merely with growing older; but now she had become increasingly concerned about the way in which she was growing old. She, like the previous worker, felt that age had crept upon her. It was with some amusement that she said, laughing:

> I really should be retiring now, although I can't think about that. I've still got a lot of life in me. But it did worry me at one time. I used to say 'Well, when I get to a certain age I'll take a few pills and that will be it'. But as I've got older I realise - well, I mean, when do you take these pills? No, it's not growing old which worries me, and dying, it's how I grow old.

50

The same worker said she had come to terms with the idea of her own death, and that this had coincided with the process of her own ageing. She had firm ideas about how she wanted to grow older, which were related largely to staying active and healthy. The concept of being in control of the ageing process was also mentioned by one interviewee, who found it interesting to compare a fit and active colleague nearing retirement age with a highly dependent resident of similar age suffering with senile dementia. She, like some other interviewees, concluded that 'Old age depends on the individual. Just how active they are, how mentally alert they are and their views on life, helps them stay young'. For another interviewee, thoughts of her own ageing were suppressed by keeping herself busy and caring for others: 'I work to lose myself'.

For all of those interviewed, working with older people in a residential home had influenced their views of their own ageing to a greater or lesser degree. The following worker felt able to use his experiences to review his personal life:

I think working here has made me more aware. The photographs in their room, seeing how they were in the past, makes me think that they too probably thought they would always be that age. It does make me think 'Where will I be, and what will I be thinking - what have I done with my life?' It has made me more aware of life in general.

This interviewee went on to say:

It has changed how I view old age. It makes you do more with your life. You can see what you should do.

Like one of the interviewees quoted above the majority said that they were more afraid of *suffering* than they were of dying, with one worker commenting 'It is the process I am afraid of, not instant death'. One worker described how working in a Home had shocked her and said 'It opens your eyes, and you think "Oh my God, I hope I never get like this" '.

Although not afraid of her own old age another worker expressed hopes 'not to have pain and disease, or be a total nuisance to everyone'. It is possible that this worker equates pain and disease with being dependant on others - she feared becoming a 'total nuisance to everyone' - but her experience of ageing had, she said, been positive so far. She felt that, while she enjoyed good health:

I don't worry about my own old age - I don't think about it very much. I think each part of life brings its own reward or its own experience. Old age,

51

in its own way, could be just as rewarding as it was being young.

For her becoming older also had many positive aspects:

I feel much better mentally at 60 than I did at 25. I used to worry sick over all sorts of things. Now I've got older - well you seem to calm down a bit. Things just pass over your head.

One interviewee felt that working in residential care was a constant reminder of the frightening things that can happen as a result of ageing. She compared herself with those working in offices. She believed that they experience the ageing process in a different way to those working in residential care:

People who work in offices - who don't work with the elderly - can walk up the stairs and get a twinge in their knees and think little of it. But if I walk up the stairs and get a twinge in the knees, I think 'That's arthritis', and it's really quite frightening. There are aspects to old age which are really quite frightening.

Her own fears of ageing were magnified by working in a residential home, and she said she was particularly 'fascinated by residents' loss of memory' which she said she found especially sad and ironic, in view of the busy lives many of them had led in the past. However, she believed that the gradual decline consequent upon the ageing process ensures an acceptance of and readiness for death. This is reflected in the following statements, each of which were said with incredulity and some dismay in her voice:

Some residents can't remember when you ask them how many children they had. And I think 'All those years, the prime time; and they used to call those children hundreds and hundreds of times by name - and now they can't even remember them'. I sometimes think 'What's life all about, when you can't remember what's happened in your life?'

I thought when you get to your 60s and 70s it was Mother Nature's way to give you arthritis, and this was to gear you up slowly and surely so that when you were going to die it is a release, and that you will actually look forward to wanting to die because you are in so much pain. I do believe that whole-heartedly, because I have seen so much of it. And I have thought 'Well, Mother Nature really does build you up slowly to that'. But I think she (Mother Nature) does go drastically wrong when she leaves you for years and years like that. That's what I'm afraid of.

6 Feelings about death and dying among residents

Feelings of attachment

Dependency relationships and past experiences of closeness

Given the high physical and emotional dependency of many residents in local authority homes for older people it was not surprising to learn that, to a greater or lesser extent, staff members became attached to the people for whom they provide care. The trigger for becoming attached to residents was different for everyone, however. For some staff, relationships based upon the dependency of residents were thought to create a closeness which replaced that of the residents' own families. One interviewee felt a deep sense of injustice when families did not visit their relative in the Home; he felt aggrieved when they had attended the funeral (especially because they had wept). For another, the Home and its residents provided *her* with a substitute family, recreating feelings of belonging and security and thus allowing her, as she reflected, to care for residents as though they were her own family.

She said how, when she was nineteen, after her mother's death, she had felt abandoned but that caring for people fulfilled this need in her. Also, she said that having had a bad experience during her mother's death she acknowledged that she had come into care work partly to lay a ghost. Previously she had thought that death was always painful and distressing, but was now searching for a contrary experience each time someone died in the Home - 'I grieve for my mother through the people here'. She felt this had been achieved and that she was more at peace with her earlier negative experiences. As a result, she described herself as lonely although she said that she could relate best to residents who had no family. She described how, to feel more attached, she had 'adopted' a resident, and that she 'felt responsible for her'. She added that when this resident died, she had: ' . . . cried for weeks; I think of them as my own mother or father'.

However, for the above interviewee, her experience influenced how she responded to the death of other residents but she stressed her need to avoid such strong feelings again: 'I learnt my lesson being close. I would never get that close again - I'd keep my distance'. But, interestingly, she concluded: 'You should not be in the job if you do not get attached'. Speaking of her first experience of death in the Home, she said:

> I was very emotional because it was the first one I had come across. I was not quite sure what to do. The bereavement was as though it was someone in my own family. It was like I had lost someone who actually belonged to me. It is like a part of you.

The need to be close to residents was a recurring theme in the interviews, with a heart-felt testimony of this being expressed by the above care assistant: 'I'm only really happy when I am at work. The reward of the job is in the kisses and cuddles'. This interviewee was the only one who continued to feel such an intensity of feelings with each death, saying: 'It does not change with time, it is like that with everybody'. However, many of those interviewed said that feelings of loss diminished as their experience of the number of people dying in the Home increased. One commented: 'When I first saw someone who had died, I cried. But you get used to seeing it and I do not get so upset now. I think "They are at rest now" '.

One interviewee felt that staff could become too emotional when a resident was dying and that this was detrimental for that resident, who should not be subjected to the strong emotions of their carers:

> Residents need to be protected from the over-emotional staff. Some are very emotional at the slightest thing, and a resident may think they are worse than they are. If someone is very ill, and they do not know when they are likely to go, if a carer is perhaps shedding a tear they will think 'It may be tomorrow' or 'It must be near because I have got an emotional carer here'. But an hour or two later another carer can go in and not be emotional, and this can be confusing.

Some believed that they could retain a distance between themselves and residents. One care assistant said that she tried not to put her 'personal feelings into it because it would not be right. Death does not bother me'. She continued: 'One dies, then it is on with the next one'.

For one interviewee it was important for her not to become involved emotionally in the lives of residents: 'You do not have to be emotionally involved with everybody. Emotions, if they come out, can destroy the person'. Nevertheless, this seemingly detached approach appeared to reflect her belief that, by seeing a care assistant being emotional, some residents would fear the worst and either become distressed themselves, or give up hope.

For most of those interviewed, being attached to residents was imbued with guilt in the sense that it was in some way 'wrong' to become attached. They felt that being attached went against the views of those who had 'trained' them (or they thought that it would not be approved of by their manager). With a sigh (and finally with a laugh) one care assistant said: 'Although you are told not to get attached, it's so hard!'. Another said: 'You do try to keep neutral, but it is not always possible to do that'. Yet another interviewee found that: 'However much you try not to, you do get attached to them; and when they get very ill, you get very choked'. A worker in another Home echoed this, saying: 'It can be distressing if you have become attached, and if you have looked after the person for a long time'.

The role of key worker

Some workers referred to the attachment, or 'closeness', which develops when a 'key worker' system operated in the Home. One care worker, for example, said:

> With the 'key worker' system you get more involved because of the total care; and if they have no family you get even more involved because you do everything for them.

Others spoke of their frustration at not having sufficient time to develop the kind of relationship they preferred with the residents in their care:

> I feel reasonably close, but it boils down to the fact that we really do not get the time for 'one-to-one'. That is the frustration of this job. You don't get the time to sit down and just chat and talk things through. I would prefer to work on a more personal level.

Regarding the nature of the attachments formed, for some interviewees there were, however, dilemmas associated with the 'key worker' system. They centred upon problems associated with 'becoming too close'. One attempted to overcome such feelings: 'You have to pull yourself away to talk to someone else'. On the other hand, another worker, who previously had worked during the night, felt that the relationship between night staff and residents was 'better' than that between day-time workers and residents because working through the night afforded more intimacy - more time was available for talking to residents: 'Some lie awake, and it is at night that their fears come out. People seem more vulnerable at night, and we talk to them'.

Individual differences among residents

What makes staff become attached to residents is different for each individual: 'You get attached in your own way to some more than others'. Another said:

> You get attached in different ways. Some like mucking about . . . and some like a fuss - you know, they like a cuddle, and you give them one. You get close for different reasons.

For one care assistant it was a particular resident's *un*popularity, with residents and staff members alike, which strengthened her feelings of attachment,

> Nobody liked her, and some were trying to get her removed. She was arrogant, but she had spirit and I liked her.

This worker considered it important to befriend this particular resident, not only because she was disliked by others but also because she had felt a deep sympathy and empathy for her (and others like her):

> They just need to know they have got a friend - that someone cares - especially if they have no relations, and especially if they are dying - even when they are the most arrogant person you have ever met . . . just to know someone is there.

Thus, interviewees often said that they became attached more easily to some residents than others. Many cited a resident's strength of character as an important component during the process of forming attachments. One care assistant was quite clear about the characteristics that attracted her to residents:

> I like the ones with spirit in them . . . those with fighting spirit. There is a lady here that I always tease in the nicest of ways. She will not go to bed until two in the morning. I make her a cup of tea and say 'Are you ready for bed?' and she says 'No, girl' and I say 'I've got a nice toy boy for you' and she starts to talk about the war, and she will have a laugh. It's so nice

because her spirit is there. Maybe to some people it's teasing, but it is not. It keeps her spirits alive.

For others communication might be minimal, yet they could still feel attached to residents. One found she could develop empathy and understanding with some residents by discovering 'small signs, which can be very rewarding'.

For some, the strength of attachment was not influenced solely by the physical dependency of residents; it was also a function of *emotional* dependency. Interestingly, mental incapacity did not seem to prevent the formation of attachment. For example, the fact that a resident had senile dementia did not necessarily impede the development of a closeness between a resident and a member of staff.

Being appreciated and reciprocity

Two additional factors were offered as important contributors to the formation of attachment, and to the development of caring relationships with residents. For some workers it was important to be *appreciated* by them. Residents who expressed appreciation to them for their care were more likely to generate feelings of attachment: 'There was one lady of 99 who was really pleased for everything you did for her, and people like that you obviously get a soft spot for'. For others, it was the *reciprocity of interest* which helped them to feel attached. For example, the sharing of family news might assist in this: 'When my daughter got married, she said "You must bring in the photos" '. The extent to which they could 'get to know' about residents - for example their background, their history, and their likes and dislikes - was, for some staff, pivotal during the formation of attachments with them:

If they have no family you get even more involved because you do everything for them. They tend to tell you little things, but there are others who want to keep themselves to themselves, and you suddenly realise you don't know a lot about them. You can't get really close to them if all you get is 'Yes' and 'No'. It is not like when somebody tells you what happened to them 20 or 30 years ago - all about their family.

'God's waiting room'

Due to the closure of long-stay hospital wards and respite beds following policy changes at the level of the local Health Trust, and as a direct result of the National Health and Community Care Act, 1990, those entering residential care usually are highly dependent, physically or mentally or both. They require more intimate care from staff than was previously the case and this influences the nature of the attachments formed between residents and staff in different ways. On the one hand the act of caring for the physical and intimate needs of highly dependant people affected the degree to which some interviewees became attached, and yet, because they said residents were dying more quickly after admission than had happened in the past, they were sometimes inhibited about wanting to form attachments with them. This could become confusing. Interviewees expressed their horror at the poor condition in which some people are admitted into residential care, both from the community and from hospital. An experienced care assistant described a resident admitted recently from hospital who was virtually comatose, and who needed constant care and attention in bed in what proved to be the last hours of her life. She was amazed that someone could be discharged in such a condition:

> They actually seem to come in dying. It looks as if the hospital needs a bed, and they actually come into us dying! - and you can see it with an experienced eye. Sometimes they have lasted two weeks here, sometimes just one night - which is very wrong. Somewhere along the line there has been a breakdown.

As a result of the intimate attachments made with residents she feared becoming overwhelmed by the amount of death occurring in the Home: 'It could take you over after a while; even more now with the clients we tend to get in here'. In an attempt to keep her fears in perspective she reminded herself that most older people remain in their own homes and that those she and others cared for in residential care were an exceptional group: 'I have a safety valve in me and I can step back and remind myself that there is only five or six percent who go into care; so there are 95% who do not . . .'

One interviewee found it a new and somewhat confusing experience when people died soon after admission because the nature and level of attachment was less clear-cut:

> If you have been looking after them a long time your feelings are a lot deeper than perhaps someone who has just come into your care, because you have not got to know them so well. But if they come in dying and you have not got to know them, it is awkward to know where your emotions are.

One care assistant was worried that soon residential homes will become more like hospitals, in the sense that residents will not be there long enough for attachments to form. She felt that, as they were likely to die sooner in the home, the ability of staff to become attached will be determined less by the character and personality of residents; in the future, she thought that the quality of the relationship would depend more upon the length of time spent by the resident in the Home. This would have consequences for the nature of the care given to the dying person:

> It was hard when a lady died very quickly because I had not got to know her, and I felt guilty. Perhaps it's like a hospice - where you just give them care - whereas in here they become like family.

Finally, one worker succinctly summed up the views expressed by some of her colleagues when she said 'This place is just a waiting room to die - God's waiting room'.

Feelings as a result of past losses

As illustrated, many thought that caring for older people in residential care produced close (and sometimes familial) relationships between themselves and residents. Additionally it emerged that some staff, whose own friends and relations had died, bring such experiences to their work with dying residents which can affect their involvement with the residents' families and with other staff. One care assistant said 'Personal experience has shown me how to handle families. I am more aware of their feelings'. For another, the experience of dealing with death and dying in her work helped her to know what to say to her own daughter when a relative died. She had talked to her, and finally had asked: 'Would you have wanted her to suffer another day - it was much nicer than seeing her struggle?' She said that the daughter 'had not thought of it like that'. For others too, the more experience they gained of dealing with death and dying, either within their personal life or in the work setting, the more they felt able to help others even though to do so could be painful: 'Everybody feels awkward about talking about death because it brings back memories'.

Feelings of past losses were related by some to the way in which bereavement was perceived. Two care assistants expressed the view that bereavement was 'self-centred'. The first said 'When people die we are ever so selfish, because we are crying because we are not going to see them again'; the second person said '. . . They've no longer got that person around. I think it's (bereavement) a selfish thing really'.

One interviewee said she had used the experience of her father's illness and subsequent death to help prepare herself for the death of residents:

Because of my experience when my dad died I can often tell when someone is going. I can tell when people are in heart failure because it is identical to when my dad died.

For one care assistant feelings of guilt persisted after she had to leave her father who had become critically ill during a visit to him abroad. She had had to return home, and he died. A tearful person throughout, she said 'Coping with death is difficult and I love them all'. She went on to explain, however, how she believed that the past need *not* be important and that she attached no significance to it in relation to her work.

The effect of her mother's death upon her work was significant for one interviewee who, for a period of time, withdrew from the work as a result:

I just could not cope with the elderly after my mother died because I thought 'Here's my mother at 45 - dead - and elderly persons of 80 and 90 still alive'. And I was angry.

But for another worker, whose family had concealed the death of her grandfather until after the funeral, it was important for her both to be with residents when they died as well as to attend the funeral if possible. She recognised that her need arose largely because she had not been able to do so with her grandfather. She added 'I lost out on my own family. There was no-one with him. I could have been with him, even though the rest of the family rejected him'.

Confused feelings as residents approached the last stages of life

Residents who expressed a wish to die

One worker compared her feelings about the death of older people with those of younger people, concluding that: ·

It's still a sad time when they die, but to me it's not as sad as seeing a young person go. When I am caring for them and they want to give up and not do anything, I can understand, because they are very tired. I may get very upset when they die, for two or three days, but I put myself back and think of all the young people who die, and that takes away that 'missing'.

One interviewee spoke candidly of her feelings of anger when older people said they wanted to die, saying:

People feel they are dead already: they don't know what they have got. I felt angry at a resident who said this because she had a lot of things. I think 'Younger people are dead' - it is not fair.

Like most, she said that she had heard many residents express a wish to die, but whilst this helped her cope with and accept their death it was also distressing for her. However, as their own age increased some could imagine how they might feel the same,

I can understand how the elderly can wish to die - how they can be so tired they want to die - through my own experience of being tired, mentally and physically. I am not yet at the stage to want to die, but can understand how the elderly could.

Not knowing what to say to residents who said they wanted to die was problematic for some, with one describing it thus: 'It's a one-way thing. You can only listen to what they repeat'. Similar feelings of helplessness distressed another worker,

The person is telling you 'I'm in so much pain, I don't want to linger on - help me' but you can't do more than you are doing. You would like to reassure them there is a possibility you could do what they are asking, but you can't and you come to a full stop. You can't reassure them.

As referred to earlier, for some staff it is particularly distressing when residents said they wanted to die; for one, sometimes this made her feel despondent about the care she was able to give them:

We try to do everything for them, but sometimes when they say that, staff feel let down and unappreciated. We take it personally. But sometimes, you think 'What is the point - they just want to die anyway?'

Another worker thought that residents who were suffering pain were more likely to express a wish to die. Through her experience she felt sure that 'You could look forward to wanting to die because you were in so much pain'. She thought that the role of staff in residential care was simply to provide rest and care for people at the end of their life,

I mean, perhaps it is the wrong way of looking at it, but I think with the elderly, they've gone full circle . . . and we are making their last time comfortable. They've had their life and they just want rest and comfort.

She believed also that the older people whom she cared for could control their time of death saying 'I think when they are ready to go, they go!' One worker sometimes was confused by her feelings in so far as she might *want* a resident not to die, but believed at the same time that it might be better if s/he did:

> I could see it as a release for them, but you don't want it to happen, although you know in some way they are not going to suffer any more.

Accepting that residents might wish to 'give up' was more difficult for some workers than others, who perhaps saw it as a failing in the care they were providing: 'I recognise the signs of death and of "giving up", but with the care that they are getting, we're not letting them give up!'. One interviewee thought that, not only was the wish to die dependent upon suffering, it was also as a result of frustration at not being able to do anything:

> People look around and see all the things they cannot do, watching life pass them by. I can understand how people can get to the point when they have just had enough. All they are doing is existing; they have no quality of life.

Another considered that when residents endured a poor quality of life then this could lead to feelings of despondency: 'It's just an existence, and death is better than mere existence because there is nothing they can do'.

Pain and suffering

A number of interviewees had formulated their own views about the ethics and desirability of euthanasia. The worker quoted above saw suffering and pain as 'pointless' and felt that to assist death for those in pain would be acceptable:

> When someone is in so much pain, what is the point? But if you really do love them, you will do what they ask you to do. How can you say it's murder when they are in so much pain?

Even though she thought her feelings might be swayed if faced with the situation herself, another was less sure however:

> The idea of euthanasia is against my religious belief but sometimes when people are suffering, I wonder. But if you see life as a series of experiences, should we be given the easy way out, of ending our lives painlessly rather than going through the experience of pain? It's all very well for me to say

that because I'm not feeling pain, but if I was having it myself I might feel entirely differently.

A thread emerged from the tapes that residents' suffering made acceptance of their death more likely - for residents and workers alike - and that this could overcome negative feelings. One care assistant described how she felt when witnessing residents suffer: 'Seeing the pain of others is painful and cruel'. Along with others, this worker had an idea about the kind of death which affected her least: 'A lovely death, a death free of suffering'. Most viewed the death of residents as a 'happy release' for them (although for those interviewed, this did not mean that they were not upset).

The process of dying

One care assistant described how she found it difficult to cope with residents who became agitated during the process of dying, stating that she felt worried when a resident became aware of his or her impending death:

> They seem to fidget and agitate. They just do not want to be there. I'm never sure whether they know they are dying or what; whether it is their bones hurting or whatever. I always hope the doctors will give them something to keep them calm.

Nevertheless, for one worker, knowing that she could be instrumental in alleviating the distress of a dying resident was a source of comfort to her:

> I sat with him and he just seemed to calm down. Up to that time he was struggling to live. You could see that he was afraid. Then all of a sudden he calmed down. It's almost as if something inside them has accepted it. Perhaps they are half on their way anyway, and it's nature's way of doing it - I don't know - but it does have a pattern to it.

Sometimes residents may cease to eat and drink. This also aroused strong feelings in some staff, who became distressed if they were asked to feed residents against their wishes. One worker thought that residents' wishes were sometimes overridden and that they should not be fed if that was what the resident preferred,

> It is a relief when they die (and they want to die) but we are prolonging their life by feeding them; even though she would push it away and say 'Why do you give me this to eat? I want to die'.

63

One interviewee described harrowing experiences of residents close to death but noted differences in individuals:

> I've heard people say 'Why am I still here, I'm no use to anyone, all I am is a burden, why can't I just go?' And there are people who cling to life, who are desperate. It does not seem to matter how bad they are. There seems to be a lot of fear attached to dying.

For one worker the 'constant illness and recovery of some residents' proved upsetting: 'It's the possibility that they are going to die - and then they recover. It's difficult because you do not know how you feel. It's like a see-saw of emotions'. This feeling of unpredictability also concerned another interviewee: 'Some struggle and recover against the odds, and others just die; but good care prolongs life, sometimes against expectations'.

One interviewee thought that some residents were more vocal than others about their feelings; and ultimately this affected her own feelings: 'Some just came out with it, and said "What is there left? I want to die" '. She began to complete the sentence with a sigh, saying: '. . . but you can't kill them, so . . .' but she never quite finished it (and looked sad).

Expected or sudden death

The degree to which staff were expecting a resident to die influenced significantly their feelings when they were dying as well as the *manner* in which the resident died. A number of staff described the way in which some residents died, in the following way:

> . . . if they are dragging on, it is sad, but in a lot of ways you are pleased because you are prepared, you know it's going to happen, and they are out of their pain.

The sight of death within the Home had left some with lasting and sad memories. One noted that, when some residents died, the pain 'passed from their face, but some were still cracked with pain', and this was upsetting for her. Another described the distress at the moment of death: 'Every individual dies differently. Some die nice and quietly but some just make a terrible racket when they go, and of course you want to do your best for these'. The enduring picture in her mind's eye was of a particular resident whose skin, upon death, had became quite disfigured. Until someone explained what had caused it she had been afraid to see residents after they had died, and this memory was still quite upsetting to her.

Different feelings were expressed about residents who died suddenly (as distinct from those who drifted more slowly towards death): 'When somebody just goes in the night, and you have been chatting with them the night before, it is more of a shock'. Although a number felt that sudden death was preferable in some ways it was harder for them to accept: 'It's sad, but nice. I'd rather someone go quick than see them suffer'. But for another worker her feelings were less clear-cut:

> There's no clear thoughts about it. Sometimes you feel it has not been fair, then other times you feel they are better off than the other person who had to lie in bed for weeks on end getting worse and worse.

Many described the shock of sudden death as being worse than the fact that the resident had died; thus, for one person, experience was important in helping her cope:

> I suppose if that had been my first one, then I would have gone to pieces; but you tend to think 'They were old, and suffering, and they are not suffering any more, are they?'

But for another, whose first experience of a resident dying was of a sudden death, it was different: 'My memory of the first person who died was of shock. It was unexpected, even though they are expected to die eventually'. One interviewee was sorry when residents died suddenly, feeling that they had missed out 'on a valuable experience'. She added,

> I had a feeling of disbelief: 'How can that happen? There are people here who are so ill, who you expect to go at any time, and yet this is the one that has gone'. It takes longer to get over it. If you have seen someone go downhill, however much you don't want them to go you are pleased they don't have to put up with any more. But when someone dies suddenly they (the residents) are cheated - have been cut off - and it seems unfair.

Helplessness

Most appreciated that part of caring for very frail older people in residential homes inevitably also means that they will be caring for people who are dying. Although one worker believed that, with the increased number of deaths she had experienced, she was able to predict death - and that this was helpful to both herself and other staff - others experienced an almost haunting sense of helplessness (referred to earlier) in their work. For one interviewee feelings of being unable to help followed her home: 'It is hard to switch off from the Home. You go to bed and it is still on your mind. You can't walk out and forget about it - it is impossible'. She continued, reflecting: 'It is a very sad thing, death, and you feel you cannot do anything for them. You can look after them, but you can't really *do* anything; you have to wait'. For some, feelings of helplessness cast doubts on their ability to care successfully, especially when a higher number of residents than usual died in a short space of time,

> It was Christmas, and we lost a lot - twelve - and it was horrendous. But when I thought about it I could see that they came in like this (*meaning*: very frail). But it does make you question your standard of care.

Similarly, for another interviewee the feeling of not being able to help lingered after the death of residents: 'You feel like you have done the job, but also you haven't done the job, and you need something to tie the two together'. This worker was referring to having something concrete to indicate that she had done the right thing for a resident who she had found difficult to help. She added,

> You go along on your common-sense, but you do not know whether you are doing the right thing; you do not know if you're speaking to people the right way. You sometimes wonder if you are treating people right.

For one interviewee her feelings of helplessness were magnified if she felt that she could not be as honest as she wished with residents about their condition,

> It is hard to remain optimistic with some of them, because you can see their point if they say they are dying, and I just do not acknowledge it. I just say what you are supposed to say.

Occasionally they found themselves in the position of 'mending bridges' for dying residents. Whilst this could be a rewarding experience, it could also make staff feel powerless. One worker described how she felt perturbed when one resident who was dying told her that she had regretted not having children. No-one had heard her say this before and, as she said: 'It was a really choking experience; it really was. Up until that point she had never said a word about it, and it was a really emotional time for a few of us'. For another, it was upsetting that she had been unable to help resolve a family rift before a resident died. She found that sometimes residents did not share their fears or worries until shortly before death. This created in her feelings of powerlessness, failure and regret:

66

You often do not know about it - the rift - until they are just about to pass away, and you don't always get there on time to contact those particular people. And perhaps, if you do, they are not interested anymore because of the years that have gone by, and they think there is nothing they can do. They do not understand how important it is to the resident.

For yet another worker it was the fear of the unknown which she found difficult 'You, as a carer, get more and more distressed because you do not know what you will be dealing with'. Many of those interviewed shared this view; others spoke about different feelings of helplessness including guilt at 'allowing' residents to be admitted to hospital where they *would* die. In one excerpt a resident on admission to the Home described to staff how deeply afraid she was of hospitals and that she would not want to be taken there when she was dying. The worker described how she had felt inconsolable when the decision had been taken out of her hands by the general practitioner who, according to her, had taken no account of her protestations to honour the resident's wishes to be allowed to die in the Home when the time came. She said:

I sometimes feel physical and emotional exhaustion, it is a mixture of both. There are so many things being thrown at you, your mind is always swimming. You want to please everyone, but you just cannot. The guilt stays with me and I feel that procedures are winning over the wishes of residents, to cover the staff.

For others too, it seemed that a resident's admission into hospital contributed to feelings of helplessness and distress; although one interviewee felt that these sentiments were not only valid, they were essential to the job: 'If I did not have those feelings there would probably be something wrong with me, or I was not dedicated to the job'.

Some staff felt that the care older people received in hospital did not compare with that given in the Home, expressing a view that some were neglected while in hospital. For example,

When she went into hospital she went right off her feet. She would not eat or drink, or walk. It was unbelievable how she had deteriorated. We feel it was neglect: she was left. The family were going in three or four times a day to give her food and drink, because it was just being left at the end of the bed. We would not have done that here. We would have fed her, encouraged her to eat.

The residents' own wishes were seen as important to another interviewee who, in recognising people's wishes to remain at the Home to die, said:

> The thing they do say is they do not want to die in hospital, they want to die here. I think that is important for us too. If we can cope and they are not in too much pain, it is important. This is their home.

Others also thought that residents became vulnerable to 'time-saving' techniques when in hospital: 'We want to protect residents when they go into hospital - against catheterisation'. Some experienced a sense of sadness and helplessness if they did not participate in the 'last offices' of residents who died in hospital:

> It's so clinical, the way they deal with them in hospital. They just plug the orifices, and that's it. It's more personal in the Home: we put a flower on the person. They are shown respect.

Some feared that residents would not be afforded the same comfort that they felt they offered in the residential home:

> It is nice when they die here really. At least you know they are not on their own. Whereas when they are in hospital they are so busy; there is no guarantee there will be someone with them. I would never want to die in hospital. In a place like this Home there is always somebody ready to sit and hold someone's hand. There is always somebody who will do that. In hospital they are always rushing up and down.

When a particular resident was admitted to hospital one interviewee overcame her feelings of helplessness by visiting regularly. However, her experience immediately prior to death has proved to be a lasting and harrowing memory for her. It was the saddest testament to the helplessness felt by many of those interviewed:

> It is important to keep contact when they go into hospital, especially if they have no relatives to visit them. Even though she was unconscious, I kissed her. When I left I asked if they would let me know when she got worse so I could go and sit with her, and I told them who I was. I went to the car and realised I had left my keys. When I went back the curtains were drawn and when I looked in they were washing her and changing her, and I think they were doing it then to save time. (*When she got back to the Home she received a telephone call asking her if she wanted to go back, which she*

presumed was because the staff thought the resident was going to die). I kept some of her things for comfort: her earrings and Rosary. I know it sounds morbid.

7 The actions of staff

The delicate dance

A feature which has been considered earlier is that interviewees often had heard residents say that they no longer wanted to go on living and that between them they experienced a range of feelings. Similarly their *actions* varied too, ranging from diverting residents from talking about the end of their life to attempting to acknowledge the resident's fears or anxieties. One recognised that staff respond in different ways:

> Talking about death and dying comes easier to some. Others turn away from it - they don't want to face it. That's their way of dealing with it. They switch off from it all together. They do not want to discuss it at all.

At some point interviewees usually said that they were faced with a dilemma when talking to residents who said they wanted to die; but for some it was more difficult to know what to do if the signal to talk was less than obvious. A complicated set of verbal and non-verbal messages appeared as steps within a kind of 'dance':

> One resident had cancer, and she knew, but she used to play a little game and say 'I'll be up walking and running before you know it' and you'd say 'Yes, of course you will', and then she'd say 'I'm only mucking about - I'm confined to this wheelchair and I'm going downhill'. When she fancied a laugh and joke we went along with her. You cannot be serious all the time, and laughing and joking for a few minutes helped her through the day. It's hard to say 'Yes, you are dying'.

As part of the 'dance' one worker described how some residents seek reassurance that they will be remembered after they have died; some referred to the need to distinguish between what style of behaviour and language to use with different residents:

> You can go into rooms in the morning and you'll have about three people say 'Oh, I wish I was dead, I didn't want to wake up this morning'. This happens regularly. I say 'Don't say that' but it depends on who it is. One resident says 'Nobody will miss me.' But I say 'I'll miss you'.

The dilemma of what to say was highlighted by another worker, who wanted to be honest and yet felt that to confirm a resident's statement directly was not appropriate:

> She said 'I'm going to die, aren't I?' I said 'Well, yes, but we all are and we don't know when. You are not very well at the moment - but we just don't know . . . ' But it's hard when you see them deteriorate before your eyes, and they are crying in pain. It is a very emotional time for the carers looking after them, let alone the person. To me, that's a truthful answer. I did not say to her that she was not going to die - and that she was going to be all right - because I did not know. Confirming what you don't know is not good.

One interviewee thought residents found comfort in her own quietness. She thought that she had learnt to pick up the signals from people if they wanted to talk, or needed to find some peace and comfort at the end of their lives:

> Sometimes when residents are poorly and are skirting around the subject, I just say to them 'Lie there quietly and I'll say a little prayer for you'. And most of them respond to that, and they say 'Thank you, I will too', and I'll say 'Well, we've done the right thing, you'll be okay'. I don't know anyone who has not responded by saying 'That's lovely, I'll do the same'. I think when people are sick and dying, even if they have not had much faith before, they are looking towards grasping at some sort of help.

For one worker it was impossible to answer such questions, and she responded in the following way: 'I'm afraid I lie to them. I don't know whether I should, but I just tell them "When the time comes, you'll know" '.

Knowing what to say - and when to say it - were matters of fine judgement for one worker, who took the lead from the resident. Others thought that, if hope and optimism were eradicated, then talking to residents about death could be destructive by diminishing the 'chance of happiness at the end of life':

I think talking depends on the people. Some don't mind talking about it and other people just don't want to think about it. It's like when people are really ill - should they or shouldn't they be told? I think that depends on the person. You can tell somebody and they could just completely give up; but with somebody else, it can give them that little bit of extra fight to keep going and they won't be beaten. If someone wants to talk to you about it then you go along and talk about it.

For one interviewee it was not only important to judge which residents wanted to talk about their future in terms of their own death; she needed also to judge whether the timing was right for a specific resident to talk: 'You have got to tread very carefully. You can try and start, but then if they don't want to talk then you cannot push it too far'. She felt that talking often was something very alien to the generation of people living in homes for older people and that this was sometimes difficult to deal with:

They are a generation which never spoke out, and our generation are used to talking (with counselling and all that) whereas for them it was a burden to bear. Sometimes they will talk, when they are down, and say 'I've had enough' but that's an end to it. Whether they feel they can't talk to us or not, I don't know.

Some took a different approach to residents who said that they wanted to die: some preferred what they described as a 'jollying-along' approach, believing that diverting their thoughts by the introduction of some activity was the best way of dealing with what residents were saying to them:

We've got one lady who says she's tired and what's the point (in living). I just say 'Oh don't be silly, cheer yourself up, it's just how you feel at the moment. You'll feel better tomorrow.' I try to rally them round - sometimes it works.

In a similar vein, some were convinced that it was not helpful for residents to dwell on death. For example: 'You change the subject. You say "Don't say that; you'll be all right" '. There were other diversionary methods used. Some attempted to reassure residents that they are not old enough to die, saying to them for example:

You are too young to go anywhere yet - you stay with us a bit longer - you could go out on a mini-bus trip. Or you see if they want to do knitting. You change the subject, try to talk about something cheerful; and they forget.

72

Some workers, on the other hand, judged how they should respond to those who said they wanted to die based on the degree to which they thought that the resident 'meant' what s/he was saying. For one worker the *validity* of the reason determined her response. She believed that residents were more likely to 'mean it' if they had 'lost a lot of their family', and therefore were very lonely, rather than that they had just had 'a rotten day'. A similar view was expressed by another, who dismissed what some residents said about wanting to die if they went on to ask for other things (if she considered such requests to be in some way 'contradictory'). For example:

> She did say that she wanted to die, but in the next breath she'd say she wanted to see her own home - she wanted to go back to London and she wanted to see her daughters.

Again for another interviewee a significant factor in determining whether a resident was 'serious' about not wishing to live was whether s/he had any family still living: 'There are some who would be better off dead, but there are others who say it who have got family . . . well, I think those people are just *saying* it'.

Similar to those who used a 'jollying-along' approach were a number of workers who said that they tried to encourage residents to view their life more positively by adopting a 'cheerful' manner. However, one acknowledged the sadness of those who said they wanted to die:

> Some just give up. They don't want to do anything. They don't want to eat or drink; it's very sad. But I say 'It's not time yet. You're not ready to go. You've got a lot of time left'. But they do get very depressed.

For another interviewee, who said she always tried to 'jolly them out of being depressed', nevertheless went on to say that 'people do eventually know they are going to die' adding that she had heard one resident saying 'I want to be in my coffin'. Then she said:

> It's terrible for them to say things like that. I've spoken to them and said 'Does it worry you if you are going to die?' and they've said 'No, it doesn't', and they are ready to go.

Not everyone thought that diverting residents away from conversations about death was necessarily a good thing. For the following worker a training course helped her to crystallise her view, and as a result she felt able to empathise with residents who told her that they wanted to die:

I did a course and we were asked if we should try to jolly people out of it. Some thought you should but I disagreed, because if I was in that sort of mood and someone tried to jolly me out of it, I wouldn't be very nice to them. If I've got the hump I like to be left alone. I think if I felt that bad, if someone said 'Never mind, you'll feel better tomorrow', I'd be really cross.

One interviewee found that sometimes residents referred to their fears in indirect ways. She believed it was necessary to interpret what they were saying in order to help them, feeling strongly that it was wrong to deny residents an opportunity to talk over their worries about death:

Sometimes they say they want to go home, and what they mean is they want to die. They elaborate on it if you ask them and they say they have had enough of it, and they want to go now.

She went on to describe what she said to residents who said they wanted to die in order to reassure them that she could help make their remaining time more comfortable:

I say 'I know it would be nice for you; I understand how you must feel, but it is not time for you to go yet. We will just try to make you more comfortable until the time comes'. I do not say to them that it's not going to happen, and I think when they see the others going they must have it on their mind. It must bring it home to them when people disappear from the scene.

The shock of the new

Emerging from the data was a sense that some people felt that they had become accustomed to dealing with death and dying, and that this familiarity provided them with important emotional protection. But most described vivid recollections of their first experience of death and dying. One worker, for example, was particularly concerned that in recounting her feelings to her colleagues she might be perceived as callous:

I was frightened with the first one, not having seen someone die before. But I got . . . it sounds hard saying 'used' to it, but it's not - I don't mean to be hard. I did not think 'Oh God, what am I going to do?' I still get upset; obviously, because you get attached to the people.

74

The above interviewee's fears perhaps were well-founded because another interviewee said that she noticed a lack of visible emotion in some of her colleagues: 'Some are very hard - *very hard'*.

After her first experiences of mortality, the implications of working with frail older people soon became obvious for one worker: 'After the first day I thought "I'm not going to cope with this" '. For another too, her first experience was both memorable and intolerable,

> The first one (who I saw die) was after I had been there for a few months and I did not cope very well. I was holding her hand when she went. Every time I closed my eyes after that I kept seeing her face, so I came out of it (the work) for a little while, and then came back. By the time I came here I was - it's a hard word to say - 'used' to it. No, not 'used' to it: I was able to 'cope' with people dying.

This distinction which she and others made - between becoming *used* to death and dying and *coping* with people dying - seemed to be important. Many felt uncomfortable that they had become 'used' to death because they thought that it did not reflect truly how they responded to death and dying. For one worker, who initially had thought that she could predict how she might feel, nevertheless experienced a wave of aftershock which had surprised her:

> Seeing someone die the first time - well I did not expect it to be okay, but it was at the time; but afterwards I realised.

Another's fears were not realised on her first experience of seeing a resident die: 'It was weird - not how I had expected it to be. It was like he was asleep'. One interviewee felt that the ease with which she had coped the first time she had dealt with a person who had died in the Home made her question the degree to which she cared for residents: 'Because I coped calmly I thought it was because I did not care very much. I don't know, even now, how I would have been if it had been someone who was close to me'.

The idea of 'coping' was a recurrent theme, suggesting perhaps that interviewees had developed skills at adapting to differing tasks within residential work with older people. For example, caring for older people in residential care ranges from sewing name tags on clothing to sitting with a person while s/he dies. One person said,

> Most care staff cope very well, except for one worker who was shocked by it (death) at the very beginning because it was the worst one she had seen. But they cope well with death as well as life - it's all part of the same job.

This same sentiment was reflected rather pragmatically by one interviewee, who said that: 'Although I was not prepared for it, it was not something that bothered me. I knew I had to do it'. A similar approach was echoed by another worker, who described death as: '. . . a process, and we just do what is necessary'. But, for another person, her first experience was redolent of what many people describe when someone dies (and what is referred to in the bereavement process as the stage when the bereaved person finds it difficult to accept the death): 'I could not believe that she was dead'.

Being there at the end

Much emphasis was placed on not leaving a dying person alone, either during the process of death or at the time of death. For example one said,

> When someone is dying you make sure there is someone there - as far as staffing allows (but they do make sure there is enough for that sort of thing). We say to the night staff when we go: 'Please don't leave them on their own'.

One interviewee continued to have uncomfortable feelings because, although she had felt it was important to be with residents when s/he died, on one occasion she had had to follow the instructions of her manager:

> My first experience was terrible. I was a raw recruit, and I knew this gentleman was dying and I just wanted to go in and hold his hand, but the Head would not let me. So I paced up and down to keep checking, without going in. And nobody was there when he died, and I thought that was dreadful. She said, 'Just leave him, there is nothing you can do for him'. I can still see that gentleman.

Sometimes being with a resident while they were dying brought interviewees into conflict with colleagues. This worker described how a lack of sensitivity displayed by her colleagues had troubled her:

> I was sitting with a lady while she was dying, and the others (staff) started mucking about. I know that the last thing to go is the hearing, so I did lose my temper, and I shoved them outside and said 'If you want to muck about, you do it outside, not in there'.

Staying with residents while they died exposed interviewees to direct questions from them. But for this interviewee, it posed few problems:

> She asked if she was dying, and I said 'Yes, but I won't leave you; you won't be on your own', and she said 'Good, don't leave me. I'm not frightened, but I don't want to be on my own'.

Whilst most did not like leaving people who were dying on their own, alone, nevertheless a tension emerged from the interviews concerning the competing needs of residents. Some felt guilty that they were rushing tasks with other residents when someone was in bed dying because they were anxious to get back to sit with him or her. On the other hand they felt guilty when sitting with a dying resident because they knew someone else in the Home might need their assistance:

> I am always rushing people. While I am giving them their tea in the dining room, I'm thinking of Elsie, alone in her bedroom dying.

Last goodbyes and 'last offices'

A strength of feeling was apparent about the need to say goodbye to residents, either before or after death. Even though a few interviewees balked at the idea of actually being present when residents died, nevertheless they felt it was important to have said goodbye, either directly to the person before death or to his or her empty room afterwards: 'It's nice to say goodbye, even though they can't hear'. But to ensure that residents were not left alone during their final days and hours some workers subjugated their own needs, possibly repressing their feelings: 'I don't like being with death but I always ensure someone is there'. One felt a sense of responsibility to make sure of this, saying: 'It is very important to know someone is with my "own" resident when she dies'.

One interviewee described how, when one resident died unexpectedly, she had felt less upset at the news because, inexplicably and unusually for her, she had made a special point of saying goodbye to her before she went off duty.

One key worker said she feels unhappy if, when she is not on duty, she is not informed when one of the residents who she works with is close to death; she preferred to have the opportunity to choose to return to work to be with the resident:

> Key workers should be involved, not shut off at the end. A lot of key workers feel they are the only one when they are on duty, but it is something which goes deeper and this should be considered.

For some, attending the funeral provided an opportunity for them to say goodbye but for those who were unable to attend, revisiting the resident's empty room was an alternative: 'I have to go in their room and say a little prayer'. For another, the funeral was a way of rounding things off: 'Going to the funeral is beneficial. It's a way of saying goodbye to them for the last time because I'm not always there when they pass away'. For another worker too, the funeral was an important aspect of helping her accept the death. She added also that,

> If I can't go to the funeral I go to the chapel of rest to say goodbye. It's upsetting at the time but it's like a chapter closed.

For some people, saying goodbye was helpful in accepting the impending death of a resident (thereby making his or her death less painful for the worker) but sometimes, the act of 'speaking' might not be in a verbal form to the resident. The following interviewee illustrates this point. He compared his feelings about two residents who had died in hospital,

> I had three favourites in the first year I came here. They all died in just over a year. They all died in hospital, but one of them I visited regularly and I could see she was just going down so I could mentally say goodbye. But the second was very sudden at the hospital. I did go to see her, but she was asleep so I never really got the chance to say goodbye, and that was worse.

Some felt it was important to make a deceased resident presentable for his or her relatives. For one, who had gone home one day and found her partner dead, having committed suicide, it was absolutely vital to her that relatives should not be subjected to what she had experienced. And, it was important for her to be able to prepare *herself* for the impending death of a resident,

> The smell of death, you cannot explain. You prepare yourself, and then you can do your job. I make them well-presented for the family to say goodbye because it is important for the family to remember how they looked - it's the last picture you take with you. I think also it is decency for themselves.

The importance of family members seeing their relative after death was also very clear for another worker, whose fiancé had died while abroad with the Army. She attended his funeral, but did not see him after his death. She had retained doubts ever since about whether he had really died, and although she said she was reconciled to it, she felt very strongly about relatives 'identifying' the dead person,

I think it is very important for the family to identify them - so they can believe they are dead. You should see them. They can see by this that they have had good care. If they don't come to see them there may always be uncertainty that the person whose funeral you have gone to is actually dead.

When a resident dies in a Home for older people it is the job of care assistants, after death has been certified, to straighten and wash the body, brush the hair, replace dentures and put on fresh clothing and bed linen. This is a task which not everyone felt they could do at first. (Although the majority of those interviewed had performed 'last offices', two had not been asked to do so). For one, the expectation proved worse than the reality, and she had felt an enormous sense of achievement when she had performed these tasks,

I was dreading it. To actually lay them out yourself is very different. I felt like I had achieved something. It prepares you for anything - now I can face anything.

But the fear of seeing the dead person prevented the following worker from ever being able to perform 'last offices':

I can't go in alone in case they make a noise. The colour frightens me; it's really on my mind all the time. I have never laid one out yet, and I don't want to.

Another interviewee felt the same:

'There's nothing to it', I was told - there's nothing to it! I could not do it because I think they can still feel. I think I'm alone in thinking this, but for me they are still there.

For one worker new to the procedure, knowing that someone was there with her who had experience was very welcome: 'The first person I washed, Alice was with us, and she said "you chat to them" - and you do'. Others described the task in various ways, but several referred to the 'strangeness' of it:

I did 'last offices' for Rose. It was a strange experience. When I was looking at her I thought I could see her breathe. I expected her to breathe.

Unlike the person in the above excerpt, another worker felt that the 'person' had very definitely 'gone': 'It's a funny feeling, they are not here anymore. You just close their eyes and wash them down'. Another interviewee also described it as the 'strangeness of the shell, the stopping of the person - they are not there anymore'. In an apologetic tone, one care assistant said that it was important to her that she ' . . . gets them all nice. Talking to them is important. I give them reassurance after death, telling them they are off to heaven'. Yet another found it helped her to imagine that the person was still alive, saying:

> You handle the person very gently because you don't realise they can't feel, so you treat them like you are just washing them. It's a strange feeling, most of the time when we do it here they are still warm and soft.

Finally, one interviewee described how she coped with performing the task by retaining an emotional distance:

> You do sort of block off when you are actually dealing with the person, but afterwards you think 'Oh, it's sad', but when you are there you are too busy doing the job. We kiss them goodbye and say our last farewell. It's afterwards that you get upset.

Talking to colleagues and friends and expressing feelings

Coping mechanisms varied. One interviewee thought that individuals had their own way of dealing with things, but did not accept that their way necessarily was right for everyone,

> If you are afraid of big emotions and exposure to feelings it must have an effect on the care they can give. 'Held back' people cannot be giving. Some people think it is best left alone, they are afraid to confront bereavement. They poke it away and can't come out with it.

She went on to say that if staff are not able to express their feelings it is, 'difficult to know how to approach people'. The value of talking to someone else was also discussed by another worker who said she had derived comfort from doing so in the past:

> It affects you in different ways. You see I'm lucky, I am a person who can talk about things. Some people can't, they bottle things up. If I am worried, I talk. I think you have got to talk about things because it helps.

Many found the support of colleagues was vital both during and after the death of a resident. One interviewee, however, thought that to give vent to feelings conflicted with her perception of her own role as a mother which she thought should demonstrate strength at all times: 'As a mother you are supposed to be strong'. For some, the expression of their emotions seemed to be dependent upon how those around them reacted; but space and time was not given over for the quiet and private expressions of grief. For example, one said,

> One lady, whose family were abroad, was dying and we told them (the family) that we were willing her to hold on until they came. But she didn't. And I was all right until I looked at the other two (workers) who were crying. I can cry and carry on with what I am doing. I don't sit down and have a good cry.

Closely related to this point was a comment made by a different worker, who considered that personal space was not possible following the death of a resident even though she felt that talking was very important afterwards. This person also reflected on the helpful effect, for her, of the research interview itself as a catalyst for the expression of her thoughts. She explained why:

> People need to talk about it. Sometimes they talk to each other, but there's not really the opportunity while you are working to talk at any great length about death and bereavement. I think it's much more beneficial to have a session like this, when we can actually have time to think about it.

Whilst some sought support from colleagues within the staff group, one considered that this was not quite sufficient: 'We do get support from each other - which is a good thing - but sometimes I think we could have a little bit more'. She went on to say that she had experienced the feeling of not knowing whether she was 'being useful', which, she thought, could have been alleviated by arranging counselling for staff:

> We are counselling *them* (the residents), but in some cases it would be nice to be counselled yourself, because you come up against some things and you really do not know if what you are saying is right. You feel it is right, but you would like someone to say 'Yes'. You need to be able to express your feelings to someone you know to say 'You are doing okay'.

The acceptance of death as 'inevitable' in a Home for older people made it possible for one interviewee and some of her colleagues to discuss the experience 'unemotionally', so she argued,

> The subject does not come up in the staff room. It's spoken about, but

there's no in-depth talk about how you feel about it. It's mentioned as a matter of fact.

The negative effects of not talking about death were reflected upon by another interviewee who regretted that staff were not encouraged to express their feelings when a resident died:

Death should not be kept under wraps - it should be talked about, however upsetting it is; it should be brought out into the open. It is when it is inside that it grows and gets worse somehow.

Another worker was convinced that the expression of emotions enhanced the relationship between herself and other more junior workers in so far as, when she became upset, they would recognise clearly that crying was acceptable - 'Whatever grade you are, I hurt if you kick me. Making it okay to cry is part and parcel of the job'.

Personal differences in what staff did in respect of showing their feelings and talking about them also were noted: 'Some won't talk to you for two or three days; others speak straight away'. Consequently, the value of a mixed age group of staff was seen as significant, in terms of the support system, because people brought their own strengths to situations. One person saw the importance of older - or at least more experienced - staff talking to younger staff:

We can offer reassurance, and make it okay to cry. Some staff talk, some do not. It's just how they are. Some of the youngsters talk quite freely. I think, with some of them, we are like their mums.

Again, for one interviewee, the support and experience of other staff helped her:

It is very hard to know what to say to reassure residents who are dying but sometimes what you may not think of somebody else will come up with, and that helps.

Nobody referred to any formalised process to explore feelings (either in groups or individually) after the death of a resident. On the contrary, they said that any expression of feelings was haphazard and dependent on what else was happening at the time: 'Talking after a death is not an organised thing, it's spontaneous'. For this interviewee the atmosphere between staff improved when a death occurred, giving her a sense of drawing together in adversity,

It is strange to see. You see them working together as a real, good team - for that time. At least it happens at the right time; when the support is needed, it's there.

Another interviewee found it sad that staff seemed only to react kindly to each other in extreme circumstances:

It's a bit hypocritical really because you don't really see the level of care between each other on a day-to-day basis until something happens, then all the staff rally round and give support.

For one, it was important that she could choose who she went to for support, and to whom she exposed her feelings: 'The comfort of friends is good but I would not wish to invoke the sympathy of strangers, people I do not know very well'. Having an opportunity to gain insight into a colleague's feelings was helpful for another interviewee because it enabled her to understand better a particular senior member of staff, whom she had perceived previously as being 'very stern': 'It was quite refreshing to think she had far more in her, and could actually tell me how she *feels*'.

For another interviewee too, the strength gained from team members was invaluable: 'If I did not talk to the team I could not cope with the day-to-day hurt and feelings we all experience'.

Some workers gained their support and comfort from their own family when a resident died in the Home. For others, humour 'back at home' played a part in helping them cope with painful feelings:

When you can't go home and laugh about it, or talk - that's when it's doing you damage and you should leave. I laugh about it after I get through the week, and I get a nice weekend off and I'm rejuvenated.

However, he was conscious of the potential for burdening friends and relatives but thought nevertheless that this was an important element in ensuring that he could continue to cope with the work:

I waffle on to my relations and my girlfriend, and to me it sounds really bad - like you have got nothing else to talk about - but it's the only way you can relieve your frustrations.

The extent to which they said they spoke to others about their experiences varied, but it seemed that the three men interviewed had an additional consideration to make when seeking someone to talk to during or after the death of a resident. Societal expectations and norms for male behaviour may preclude them from some of the support systems available to women workers: if 'men don't cry', consequently they may be unaccustomed to expressing their feelings. However, one of the men seemed to find little difficulty in coming to terms with the twin pressures of being in a caring profession, where one's feelings are exposed, and maintaining credibility with his male peer group in his private life. He said at one point 'They are all interested to know what it is like when people die - you know, what happens. . .' He went on to explain that he was keenly aware of the potential for ridicule by his friends outside of work who he thought might not understand the emotions aroused by such intimate work with dying people; but he said he felt he was 'a brave person', who resisted the temptation to repress his feelings:

> You can keep that macho stuff! It's supposed to be macho to keep it all in - but you can keep all that. They say you are not a man if you cry, but you are. I don't care. If something upsets me, I show it.

One assistant considered it therapeutic to talk with family members when her mother had died, and said that she had carried this experience into her work,

> It's much better to talk about it. When my mother died both my sisters and I could not stop talking about it. We went over, under and through it - going over it, discussing all the details of what happened and how we felt.

She went on to suggest that, although this would be good practice for staff following the death of a resident, she felt that the pressures of the job did not allow for it to occur.

. . . And life goes on

Having held the hands of dying residents, said their goodbyes and performed 'last offices' for them, those interviewed described what then faced them. Some had strong feelings about the way in which they felt that death was managed in their Home. They felt dissatisfied with, what one described as, the 'secrecy surrounding death', which she considered to be unnecessary,

> Residents are not oblivious to what goes on. When they are well and they come in to the home, they come in through the front door. When they die, I think they should go out through the front door. They come in the front door, they should go out the front door. Death is concealed in a lot of

Homes and I feel it should not be. Residents know some day they are going to die, and I don't think death should be covered up in the way it is in our Home.

What the other *residents* were told varied after a death had occurred. Some felt that the residents should always be told: 'Perhaps residents can deal with their emotions better if it is not concealed, if it is out in the open. Staff could deal with it better as well'. And, sometimes, concealing news caused added complications to an already potentially distressing situation,

> Because it is concealed here you've got to be careful what you say to certain residents. All residents should know because then you can counsel them. We have to think all the time now - 'We can tell that one' or 'We can't tell this one'.

For another person, the way residents see death handled in the Home determines how they themselves will be treated 'when their time comes'. Also they will form an impression of their own worth from what they are told when other residents die:

> It is a care assistant's role to talk to residents about their friends who die. We know how they will react, and you can do the grieving with them. One resident really felt for somebody and she went through the grieving process, and we were actually there to help her through it rather than concealing it. But that particular resident was only told because she had all her faculties. But it should be for all residents, not just for one. They all know, although they might not all say. They all know when someone is not there who should be. They should be told if someone has passed away.

Not only did they express their sadness at having to cope with death in the home, it was also the sadness of other residents which upset them, although some gained confidence from some of the more matter-of-fact ways that some residents deal with the death of others. For example,

> Sometimes they'll ask, and we'll tell them, and they say, 'Shame . . . what time is tea'. But they are all looking at the empty seats and wondering who will be having that chair next. But they do get upset if it's special friends.

One worker felt that she had borne the brunt of a resident's anger at not being told of the death of a particular resident,

We had been asked by our superiors not to say anything - and we did that - but when it comes down to the resident, if they blame anybody it will be the care assistant. She will say 'I'm not talking to her any more'.

A small number said that the way residents who had died were treated from the time of death to their removal from the Home affected how *other residents* coped with death and dying. The secrecy and the complicated arrangements which are performed when a body was removed are distressing, and affected one worker:

When someone is taken away by the undertakers, all the remaining residents are moved away from the windows. The trolley goes down the path, so if they haven't seen the black bag they might have seen the trolley and the black van anyway, so they know someone has passed away. Staff try to conceal the fact by taking the residents away from the windows near the area. If they ask, we just say 'We are moving you into the main lounge just for a moment'. A member of staff is 'put on the door' so no-one can walk through.

Pausing, the interviewee then said 'It's hard - it's so hard'. She added that she believed that residents know what is 'going on' and that as a result she finds it harder still to cope with: 'They must think that's the way they are going'. For some, the memories of particular residents linger on, and certain rooms become synonymous with them: 'Even though they have died we still call number five "Amy's room" and one particular sitting room "May's room" '.

Finally, sometimes residents were not allowed to attend funerals because it would not leave enough staff to work in the Home. This perturbed one worker:

They should be able to go to the funeral. Residents are not asked if they would like to go. It's a shame because it could be their last goodbye. They do not get that chance. They are told they are ill, but that's it. Only if they have got their 'marbles' are they told they have passed away. It's like they open the door here and say 'That one's gone, shut the door'. I feel very hurt for some of the residents that this is the attitude here.

Part Three
TENSIONS AND DILEMMAS FOR PRACTICE

'How hard and painful are the last days of an aged man! He grows weaker every day; his eyes become dim, his ears deaf; his strength fades; his heart knows peace no longer; his mouth falls silent and he speaks no word. The power of his mind lessens and today he cannot remember what yesterday was like. All his bones hurt. Those things which not long ago were done with pleasure are painful now; and taste vanishes. Old age is the worst of misfortunes which can afflict a man'.

Anon

8 Accepting death and dying and forming attachments

Accepting death and dying

Societal messages about usefulness and social loss

Generally speaking the death of a child or person considered to be in their 'prime' of life is seen as being more tragic than the death of older people. However, different values are placed on an *individual older person*, whose loss to society upon death may be determined largely by their usefulness to that society: the larger society - the world, their country or the community in which they have lived - or to a smaller community, for example, if the person has lived in a residential home for older people. The death of an elderly world leader, artist or politician attracts emotional plaudits from the media, with lengthy expositions describing their contribution to society. This may seem self-evident, but it may also reflect a more subtle societal message that goes beyond mere recognition of talent: older people may be considerably more valued if they continue to *contribute* something to the community. This is similar to Glaser and Strauss' concept (1967) of 'social loss', which they found was a key determinant of the quality of care given to dying patients.

Great importance is placed upon people 'keeping in touch' with the world and 'staying young': often older people are described as being 'wonderful' if they can maintain attributes associated with youth. Millions of pounds are spent each year on staving off the effects of the ageing process.

The media tends to compound negative stereotypes of old age by presenting older people as 'miserable', 'ugly', 'complaining', and 'burdensome'; often they are portrayed as being alien to the world they inhabit and are described in patronising or angry tones, for example, 'crinklies', 'wrinklies', 'past their sell-by date' and other such offensive terms which, if applied to other oppressed groups, would be condemned as discriminatory. Perhaps individuals in society do not want to be reminded of what may lay ahead and rather than preparing the foundations for a more tolerant attitude to those who become physically or mentally frail in old age, they end up by ridiculing and deriding them.

So, arguably, many of those who die in old age are not mourned by society: it acknowledges that death is inevitable in old age, but perhaps too readily 'forgets' the life of the older person. Similarly, it is the *process* of dying which many people do not find acceptable, and this may add to our understanding of why the care of those aged over 75 still remains a key responsibility of institutions, including residential homes. But Fox questions the suitability of such Homes in providing care for vulnerable and sick people. The author believes these institutions to be '. . . oddly unsuited organisationally to its enterprise', and is concerned that 'vulnerable sick humans are drawn into monolithic organisational arrangements by which they are to be cured or cared for' (Fox, 1993).

The broad societal acceptance of the death of *older* people may be reflected within residential homes, although little recognition seems to be given to the effects on the staff working in them. It was claimed that those entering local authority residential care in the Homes studied are likely to die within six to twelve months of admission, and will need a high level of personal and intimate care during that time. It is also evident that residents are less likely to be admitted to hospital prior to death than those living in the community and that they will be cared for within the Home until they die.

Unlike most of us, those working directly with very old people are confronted daily with their own ageing and mortality. Most of those interviewed related 'old age' not in chronological terms, but in relation to the effects of physical or mental frailty. Because they were not thought of always as 'old', if a resident died suddenly the loss was often considered to be greater.

The process of death and the nature of relationships

One feature emerging from the analysis of the interviews was that when a resident declined slowly towards death acceptance seemed greater (although this may not necessarily be a predictor of the degree to which the person is mourned). Generally speaking when this 'slow-motion' death occurred those interviewed felt that it better prepared them for the death of a resident, and therefore they found acceptance easier. Also, the nature of the relationship appeared to influence significantly the level of acceptance, almost as much as the way in which the person died. Some interviewees experienced a confused set of emotions, between feelings of relief that the resident was no longer suffering, to feeling powerless that their role in the system prolonged suffering. And for some, acceptance was impeded by a sense of guilt: they felt impotent to relieve the stress or pain in those they cared for, and experienced a sense of failure if a resident was removed to hospital to die.

Acceptance of the death of residents also seemed to be related to a principle of 'fairness': if someone is old, suffering, and has 'had their life', then it is more acceptable that they die. And yet there are subtleties within this conception. As already mentioned, if someone dies suddenly, without first having suffered an illness or slow deterioration, then acceptance of a resident's death may be more difficult for the worker. A sense of disbelief also seems to contribute to a non-acceptance of death. Feelings of uncertainty may follow, which can confuse staff further. As the psychoanalyst Langer pointed out, 'Man can adapt himself to anything his imagination can cope with; but he cannot deal with chaos (Langer, 1960, p. 287).

Religious beliefs and the ability of staff to relieve suffering are influential factors, it seemed, in determining the degree of acceptance among those interviewed. For those with religious beliefs tensions and dilemmas abounded. In some cases their experience with people who were dying caused them to question the existence of God, but often they concluded that it was the medical profession, and themselves, who were responsible for the prolonged suffering. For some, the notion that death came as a relief to the sufferer sometimes did little to promote feelings of acceptance.

For many of those interviewed, their acceptance of the death of residents was influenced by their personal experiences. Most of those who had someone close to them die, and whom they considered to have been 'too young to die', seemed more accepting of the death of residents. However, it was apparent that some showed a dulling of affect, leading to a diminished level of sensitivity, which it is possible to interpret as a defence mechanism. Whilst it is clear from the literature that many writers believe health workers *need* to develop defence mechanisms it is also argued that self-awareness and insight are important contributors to the delivery of appropriate physical and emotional care to dying people. Thus, if staff do not recognise the significance of personal experiences in their work they may become overwhelmed and suppress or ignore painful feelings. This is likely to affect both their work and their personal lives. Adjustment to the death of younger friends and relatives is seen as vital for all helping professionals, but perhaps this is especially true for residential workers. If they express or harbour resentments about caring for people who often say they wish to die, or who feel 'ready' to die, it is likely to affect their ability to provide appropriate care.

Working within a residential setting engenders confusing and conflicting feelings for staff and this was apparent for most if not all of those interviewed:

whilst they acknowledged death to be a natural event, and accepted the readiness for death of residents who were suffering, they felt unprepared for the emotional effects of caring intimately for people during their final months of life.

People who do not work in this environment rarely need to consider existential questions of death in such depth and with such frequency. Residential staff are attempting to marry the norms of society, which tend ideologically to accept or even 'welcome' death at the end of a long and useful life, with their experience as workers, which requires them to accept death - and thus *loss* - among those to whom they have become attached during the course of their work. The act of balancing good and sensitive care for older dying people with the need to protect oneself from overwhelming feelings is not an easy task.

Forming attachments

Attachments between adults in residential homes

In a recent book on attachment Howe (1995) makes three claims early on:

(i) The kind of person or 'self' we become forms and arises in social relationships; (ii) the type of self which forms depends largely on the quality of those social relationships; and (iii) the way the self handles present social relationships, depends on the self's experiences of past social relationships. (Howe, 1995, p. 2).

In the main, most writers on attachment consider the phenomenon mostly in relation to social relationships formed during the early years of life. Yet in the present study many of the interviewees spoke at length about the way in which attachments formed with older people during the later stages of life were of importance too.

There are a number of factors which contribute to the forming of relationships and attachments between residents and staff. On entering care many losses are experienced by older people: they lose their home and most of their personal belongings accumulated over many years; they may lose contact with friends, neighbours, carers and home care workers; even their family may not visit regularly after they enter residential care. Increasingly admission is precipitated by a crisis and there is little time in which to plan the move into care. They may leave their home unexpectedly, never to return again. Often, therefore, they enter care in a highly vulnerable state and it is to staff that they will often turn for comfort and a sense of security.

But it is not only residents who are susceptible; staff too may have a need to form relationships or attachments with those for whom they care. But there are dangers. The nature of the relationship between qualified professionals and their clients is a feature of the formal training of medical staff and social workers and they are expected to explore fully the possible implications of becoming too attached. However, this is not generally the case within residential work. Relatively few staff attend only the most basic of courses, which usually address the more practical aspects of care work. It was apparent from this study that there exists considerable confusion in the minds of staff about their role in the lives of those for whom they care: they know that they become attached (to greater or lesser degrees) to residents but invariably believe this to be wrong. Some said that their managers (and some trainers) may have 'warned' them of the dangers of becoming attached, and yet many face a dilemma because they believe it is an inevitable and vital part of their job to do so. From a psychoanalytic perspective, the potential is great for transference and counter-transference to take place between worker and resident; indeed a number of interviewees referred to residents as being substitutes for their own mother or father (who had died).

On the other hand, staff who did not experience or express feelings of attachment often said they were perceived as 'cold' or 'unfeeling' by their colleagues. But being 'upset' about the death of a resident was seen by many as a weakness, and yet the same people often saw it as inevitable if they are doing the job 'properly', thereby producing another tension and dilemma for staff.

There is often a duality or reciprocity in the attachments formed in residential care. As mentioned, the emotional needs of staff too are part of the dynamic. It is often argued that if staff become appropriately emotionally attached it is possible that the care they provide will be of a higher standard, but the effects on the staff member when residents die might then be felt as strongly as if it had happened to a member of their own family. Also, repeated bereavements could incapacitate the worker to such an extent as to prevent them from working effectively.

If attachment is considered a 'good' thing for the quality of care for residents at the end of their lives then the support mechanisms and training of staff will, it is argued, need to be at a similar level of intensity as that provided for health care workers in hospitals and hospices.

It is possible that those who do not form attachments with residents, perhaps appearing to favour a more distant approach, may be motivated to do so not because of a lack of sensitivity but as a form of defence against the inevitable feelings of loss when residents die. Interviewees often said that they feel unprepared for the task of caring for very frail, dependent residents; and they anticipated that support will be limited or not available at all. As a consequence, to help counter feelings of attachment it is possible that they will tend to infantilise and patronise residents. But such reactions could be seen as a subconscious form of defence against powerful and painful feelings. The act of infantilising residents may make it more acceptable to the worker to clean up faeces and dribble, for example. Similarly, calling residents 'girls', 'pet' and 'dearie' may contribute to a process of de-sensitisation which helps workers to distance themselves from the emotional effects of becoming attached whilst at the same time creating an illusion of intimacy. Thus it may serve to *de*tach staff, ultimately from the death of residents. But the implications of such a pool of suppressed feelings could be considerable in terms of the well-being of staff and, in turn, for the care of residents.

Gender issues

The workforce of carers in homes for older people traditionally has been drawn from women, many of whom have family commitments which necessitate them being at home at key times of the day; often it is the opportunity for part-time and shift work which is particularly attractive to them. However, the level of unemployment has opened up this work to men who in the past tended not to consider care work as an option. Male carers are forming a small but significant part of most staff groups in residential homes.

From the interviews it emerged that they soon came to appreciate that the occupation is quite unlike most others: residential work offers potential for making relationships and forming attachments with those for whom they care, and from the interviews it was apparent that this was sometimes a shock or revelation to them.

Gender issues concerning the formation of attachment to residents also constitute another tension within practice. Although only three men were interviewed the implications of some of their experiences may apply more generally to male carers in Homes. Some of the men interviewed expressed surprise at their own feelings about particular residents (both male and female). They said that they had been unprepared for the nature of the work, not in the physical sense but in so far as they had not expected that they would become 'close' to residents. Although many of the women interviewed expressed their reluctance to show emotion when a resident died most thought that, if they *had* cried, they would have gained the empathy and support of their colleagues. However, this was not the case with two of the male carers, who saw mourning as a 'selfish' activity. Interestingly, however, another male care assistant claimed to have overcome some of the socially constructed expectations of male behaviour and he said he felt proud that he could express his feelings.

Although men joining the nursing profession is not new, the rise of males entering the caring professions is uncharted territory. Thus, it is important to recognise any specific aspects about the 'male' repertoire of characteristics within the care setting from the residents' point of view. Perhaps, for some older people, it will be important to help male staff to remain 'male', while still exploring ways for them to show their feelings towards residents as well as to discuss them with their colleagues. It is interesting to note that a number of authors conclude that boys appear to be more vulnerable to the effects of severed attachments than girls (Bowlby, 1979; Hetherington, 1980). If it were the case that men too are more vulnerable than women, then coupled with society's expectations that they should be 'brave' and not 'cry', the implications for their emotional well-being as male carers could be profound.

The changing nature of the job

The nature of residential care for older people is changing rapidly. Dependency levels remain high, yet the staffing ratios to cope with high dependency generally are low. In addition, the rate of death in the Homes studied was said to have risen over the past two years. The implications of this for the formation and nature of attachments between residential workers and residents are significant. In the past staff came to know about the biographies of residents through talking to them over many months or even years. Staff, too, shared stories about their own families: for example, they would take in photographs of weddings and Christenings to show residents. Intimacies were exchanged, and they got to know what pleased individuals. It is conceivable that the increased physical care required now could lead to the creation of more rapid attachments between workers and residents; but it is also possible - and, it is argued here, probably more likely - that staff will be *less* willing or able to form attachments with people they know will die soon.

Finally, it will be remembered that all of those interviewed felt it was imperative that a dying person should not be left alone. However, with the increasing number of deaths in residential care the call on both the time and the emotions of staff may become untenable. Again, this knowledge may dilute the strength of attachment which care assistants are prepared to make with residents.

9 The value of talking and aspects of the environment

The value of talking

Talking: to whom and about what?

The therapeutic effects of talking about inner feelings are accepted almost as a self-evident truth, as are the dangers of not doing so. Nevertheless, it is worth wondering why so many people seem to find it difficult to do? It is often with consummate ease that we encourage staff, almost without question, during training sessions to 'Talk about something which means a lot to you', despite the fact that many seem to find it a difficult and alien experience. And the paramountcy of women in the caring role - as daughter, wife or mother, or combinations of all three - may well encourage the deferment of the *expression* of emotion.

With regard to staff generally, three distinct themes were apparent from the analysis of the interviews in relation to 'talking'. Firstly, there was what staff felt it was acceptable to talk about *with residents,* regarding illness, death and dying; secondly, what staff said to *each other* about death and dying among residents in the Home; and, lastly, what they said to their own *friends and family.*

Talking to residents about death and dying

As we approach the later stages of life, social networks and contacts diminish and conversation becomes more difficult to accomplish. Many older people who live alone find it difficult to converse; many have lost touch with events in the outside world. Older people are confined, largely as a result of poor mobility and increasing social and physical isolation. Thus, any of the potential benefits of talking about feelings and experiences may be less available to many older people.

Nowadays when people enter residential care it is likely that they will have lived alone for some time and that they will enter care in an extremely frail condition. They are likely to have become unaccustomed to talking to people, and it is important therefore that the institution does not present the new resident with a 'culture shock', in which they are expected suddenly to reveal their innermost feelings as soon as they come into the Home.

The ability of staff to talk to residents about their wishes when they die, or about their impending death, seemed to depend not only upon their relationship with them; it was also a function of the culture and management style of the Home. Care assistants in general may lack the confidence to deal with residents' fears or wishes because they think they do not have the 'authority' to do so. Among those interviewed, they believed this was the job of a more senior person (even though some said they felt capable of doing so themselves). They confided that they did not always inform an officer when a resident wanted to speak about his or her condition; and they were unsure whether, if they had, that the officer would have spoken with the resident. If less experienced staff lack the confidence or ability to ask these questions then arguably residents are less likely to receive the appropriate emotional care and support at the end of their lives. And if residents are asked to wait to talk to someone more senior, some will feel rejected and others that they are a nuisance to staff and then repress the subject.

Recognising that some residents need or want to talk about their impending death is not the same as saying that all people who are dying want to talk; but only a skilled worker can recognise the difference. However, giving the 'wrong' messages - for example, by saying how busy one is - could discourage residents from raising the topic.

Making general assumptions and applying them to all situations is usually ill-advised. The old war-time slogan 'Careless talk costs lives' is recalled because of the connection between its original intention and the possible detrimental effects of 'off-the-cuff' or ill-considered comments to residents. Many interviewees referred to 'jollying-along' residents whom they perceived as becoming maudlin, morose or depressed. But perhaps the resident would have called their behaviour contemplative, thoughtful, or just plain 'being quiet'.

Finally, the use of reminiscence and recall work with dying residents may be therapeutic for some and yet quite destructive for others. Thus the balance of knowing which residents to talk to, and when, is a fine one. Neither innate ability nor training alone is likely to produce the preferred outcomes.

Talking to each other

It seemed important for staff to be able to talk to each other about their experiences, on the grounds that it was only their colleagues who will have known of their involvement with the resident and who would be able to relate closely to them. The degree to which staff actually talk to each other varies, possibly because, for them, the therapeutic effect of doing so is unclear or unproven. The potential is there for an enhanced feeling of team-spirit and understanding, and yet rarely was this referred to by those interviewed. When it happened, interviewees valued it greatly and it tended to strengthen their commitment.

Assuming that a connection is sustainable between talking about feelings and improved care to residents then if this potential is lost, because staff are not given the time to exploit their mutual support networks, then the cost on the emotions of staff would be high. Furthermore, a danger would exist that any repressed emotions would serve to harden their future resolve *not* to be affected by subsequent deaths. These are compelling arguments - which to some extent were validated in this study - but they have not been substantiated conclusively by other research findings. It may be acceptable, however, to assume that there is a connection between staff talking about their feelings and the effects upon resident care until it is contradicted. And, arguably, the extra demands placed on residential staff by virtue of the increased frailty of residents may make it more important to talk than ever.

Talking to friends and family

Thirdly, although the value of talking to friends and relatives should not be minimised, the limitations of doing so ought to be acknowledged. From the interviews there emerged issues of confidentiality, as well as some care assistants not wishing to 'burden' people outside of the work-place with their worries. Most recognised these dilemmas, but rather than talking solely to their colleagues they decided often that it was best not to talk to anyone. Again the inherent danger of this is that staff will repress their feelings completely and may become so accustomed to doing so that they will think it is the best way of coping.

Talking as catharsis

Finally, talking, it is argued, assists in the process of adaptation of staff to their situation and as a consequence they need an opportunity to do so when dealing with residents who are dying, who may seek comfort and guidance from their carers. But staff also need to talk about their own feelings, about the pain and suffering they witness. A tension is ever-present for them: between knowing that a resident will die quite soon and the knowledge that if they talk to residents when they express fears then this will create a special bond between them, the result of which may be considerable distress for the carer when the person dies. Therefore it is seen as vital that residential workers are actively encouraged to talk about these tensions, to acknowledge them and to adjust to changing situations. One way to achieve this aim might be for them to see that consulting the staff counselling service is not a failure, and does not imply that they cannot cope with the work. On the contrary, seeking help could be seen as a sign that they have the insight to want to talk about their feelings.

Aspects of the environment

The relationship between care and the environment

The environment of homes for older people - the 'circumstances, objects, or conditions by which one is surrounded' (Longman, 1987) - significantly affect the quality of the experience of death and dying, both for those who work in them as well as for those who will die in them. It is not only the physical structure, decoration and location of the building which insinuate themselves on the character of a Home, but also the routines, activities, appearance and attitude of staff - as well as the overt 'purpose' of the Home; all have an impact.

At the time of this research few of the Homes had been upgraded to meet with registration authority requirements. The consequence is that many include: rooms which have multi-occupancy; long narrow corridors; poor bathroom and toilet facilities; and large lounges and dining rooms. They were designed for residents who were ambulant and who were unlikely to spend all day within the confines of the establishment. However, this is no longer the case. Currently high (and rising) dependency levels, coupled with low staffing ratios, militate against the creation or maintenance of links with the community outside the Home and this in turn is likely to foster an institutionalised culture. Most new admissions to the residential homes in the study were above 80 years of age and therefore family and friends may themselves be quite elderly. Consequently, the potential for residents receiving visitors decreases, as does the likelihood of being taken out of the Home for visits. Social isolation and an institutionalised atmosphere can be compounded by services visiting the Home (see Tobin and Leiberman, 1976) - such as doctors, community nurses, dentists, opticians, chiropodists and library facilities - and thus minimise the need to leave the building. The significance of these factors may be that residents become disconnected with the world outside the walls of the Home. On the one hand this may allow them the peace to consider the end of their life, and to prepare for it, but, on the other, it may alienate or depress them to such an extent that they have a real desire to die, although in different circumstances they would not have expressed such a wish.

Within such an environment it could be argued that residents are more likely to achieve the kind of death which historically has been labelled the 'good' death i.e. a slow decline and controlled retreat into death. However, it is considered unlikely that such an institution would either be conducive to the free expression and recognition of feelings and emotions of the residents, or capable of nurturing compassion and a genuinely caring attitude among the staff who work in it.

In respect of the experience of caring for residents who are dying, the environment of local authority residential care homes is full of tensions and dilemmas and to many it is confusing. It is called a 'Home', and in the sense that it is a place where people stay and live it does in some respects resemble 'home', but, by the very nature of the work undertaken in residential homes, the environment and routines tend to prevent the full expression of choice to residents. That staff wear uniforms may reinforce the impression of the establishment as being somewhere where people are 'sick', and where medical expertise might be available. This is far removed from most metaphors of 'home' or 'homely'. Expectations are raised about the nature and perhaps the quality of care by such symbols.

Routines contribute to the environment of residential homes, one of these being the issuing of drugs, usually three or four times a day. During 'medication rounds' drugs are administered from a locked trolley and recorded on a formal document. Other routines serve to add to the institutionalising effects of residential care. Bath times often are dependent upon whether staff have the time to help (rather than when a resident might want to take one). Records are kept of behaviour, sleeping and eating habits, as well as whether the bed had been wet or soiled during the night. Usually, none of these practices are present when a person lives in the community, so, again, the resemblance to a 'home' is somewhat tenuous.

God's waiting room . . . ?

There is some evidence from what interviewees said that staff and residents alike recognised that the move to residential care represented the place where they would die (with one describing it graphically as 'God's waiting room'), and yet, in the main, this was something that was referred to rarely. It is not yet the case that the care of older people who are dying in residential homes is seen as the daily business of staff working in them as it is of those in hospitals and hospices, the environment of which is concerned overtly with the care and comfort of the dying. Anyone entering the hospice system is in no doubt that they are soon to die, but this allows those around them to respond accordingly. Patients will choose whether they want to be helped to come to terms with death and every effort is made to create a conducive environment for this to occur. Patients in the care of a hospice can be reasonably confident that their pain will be responded to quickly and effectively by qualified practitioners. Usually, trained social workers are available to counsel patients, relatives and staff alike, and such support systems often are quite sophisticated.

It is acknowledged (see Clark, 1993, for example) that there is an overlap between palliative care and chronic disease - in the sense of not necessarily treating patients in order to cure them - and that there are variations between the locations in which it is provided. As already argued, the care of older people in residential homes is more concerned now with the care of chronically sick people who quickly fall into the category of requiring palliative care, even though it is said that often there is difficulty in defining an exact time when one transfers to the other (Clark, 1993). In a recently published Health Trust's Annual Plan within the authority studied, palliative care is defined as 'total care when the disease is not responsive to curative treatment'. As most recently admitted residents - and existing residents - might be said to fall within this definition, then the pressures upon staff are likely to be significant.

Conclusion

If there is such confusion about the task of residential care then it is perhaps not surprising that care workers themselves are troubled by the marked change in some of the tasks which they find themselves employed to perform. Many feel torn between conforming to an unsaid rule that the subject of death is to be glossed over with residents - and often between themselves - and the nagging feeling that many would welcome an opportunity to talk about their thoughts and feelings on the matter. In addition, they often have to cope with powerful emotions, for example about not wanting to leave residents alone while they are dying. Facing such dilemmas and tensions places enormous stresses upon staff, who may not always be confident of support from their managers. To compound this further, they are left largely alone in their dealings with residents and yet fear that they will face criticism if they step over an invisible yet moving boundary. Also, if, by the culture of the Home, staff are restricted to the provision of basic physical care then considerable potential might be lost. But the sting in the tail is that by encouraging staff to recognise and confront issues of death and dying, unless they are given training coupled with support during the process, then residents and staff alike may suffer adversely.

A degree of insight into the ageing process may be a necessary prerequisite to empathising with an old and dying person, but certainly compassion alone may not be enough to help an older person die at peace. Although many of those interviewed felt that care staff needed a 'natural' ability to be successful carers, most recognised the benefits of training and good support systems. Without such support some of the consequences could be worrying: for example, it seemed that some staff could be censured by colleagues if they were 'over-emotional', and that sometimes this was considered a sign of weakness.

Most of those interviewed said they felt unprepared for the emotional impact surrounding the care of dying people. The implications of this no doubt will be of concern to policy makers and managers, both in the sense of developing

102

appropriately planned resources for the growing older population and in respect of their human resource (HR) strategies. Many staff hours in residential care already are being lost through staff sickness. It is not possible without detailed research to predict how much of this is due to stress or exhaustion. But anecdotal evidence gleaned from the interviews indicates that a number of staff remain after their normal working hours when a resident dies. Those interviewed often referred to having difficulty in 'getting on with the job' after the death of a resident to whom they had been close, and that they 'carry it with them'. If this continues to be the case, even though in the future the time to make relationships might be even more foreshortened than at present, then the rising number of people who die in Homes is likely to have serious implications for the health and well-being of staff. The benefits of 'professionalising' staff could minimise these effects to some extent but, arguably, by doing so the nature of residential care could become over-medicalised.

Generalising findings from a small-scale qualitative study to the wider community of residential provision is not possible. The aim of this book, and of the research, has been to explore the experiences of residential carers, and to highlight some of the tensions and dilemmas which emerged from in-depth interviews with twenty people working in five local authority Homes for older people, all of whom care regularly for residents who are dying. Perhaps unsurprisingly those interviewed spoke a great deal about their feelings. A reminder of the power and depth of those feelings is made at this point, the following twelve short excerpts serving as examples:

When I was a child . . . death seemed so far away, and I was just afraid; I've just always been afraid

I grieve for my mother through the people here

I cried for weeks; I think of them as my own mother or father

Coping with death is difficult . . . I love them all

I couldn't cope with the elderly after my mother died; I was angry

You . . . get more and more depressed because you do not know what you will be dealing with

We put a flower on the person. They are shown respect

I kept some of her things for comfort . . . I know it sounds morbid

It's hard to say 'Yes, you are dying'

I'll say a little prayer for you . . . 'Thank you, I will too'

I did 'last offices' for Rose. It was a strange experience: I half expected her to breathe

It's hard - it's so hard

Similarly, the following adjectives appeared in Part Two and capture the power and range of those feelings:

awkwardness	fatalism	peacefulness
optimism	powerlessness	helplessness
sadness	fear	fascination
distress	pain	injustice
rejection	loss	selfishness
frustration	guilt	inhibition
intimacy	sorrow	agitation
reconciliation	vulnerability	despondency
shock	failure	regret
repression	morbidness	loneliness
grief	melancholia	detachment
achievement	reassurance	anger
respect	depression	attachment

Left to fester, the more negative feelings are likely to affect the care of residents. But brought to the surface and given expression in a bureaucratic manner could lead to even bigger problems.

As more highly dependent people are entering residential care nowadays then there is a greater likelihood of such Homes becoming more like hospitals and nursing homes. The implication of this is that staff will have to face death in others more often and as a consequence they may become immune, thus affecting their relationships with residents. If this were to be the case then the chance of people dying being 'accompanied' - seen by Seale (1995) as a key task of carers - may be limited.

We have seen that the experiences of staff when caring for people in the later stages of life are affected by many factors and that the way in which they are supported seems to be a crucial feature in the equation. A publication in May

104

1995 by 'Counsel and Care' called *Last Rights* contains the following poignant statement . . .

> Death is rarely joyful, and dying in a home can be a particularly melancholy business. Retreating from one's own home and loved ones to an anonymous establishment is a poor prelude to the last days of life, a time when almost everyone wants to be surrounded by familiar sights and sounds and by loving and well remembered friends and relatives. To meet one's end without such comfort is the ultimate loneliness. (Counsel and Care, 1995, p. 1).

It would appear that those interviewed experienced their role as wanting to offer some of this comfort to those for whom they provided care but that they were prevented from doing so, sometimes by factors outside of their control and sometimes because they were simply not sure about the best way in which to care. And so their best intentions often were punctuated by questions such as 'Should I talk about death to the resident?' 'Do *I* broach the subject or do I wait for them?' or 'Should I talk to others about my feelings - and is it acceptable to *have* such feelings?' Perhaps a good place to begin to support staff is to start by discussing some of these questions openly.

Bibliography

Ariès, P. (1981), *The Hour of our Death*, Peregrine Books.

Ariès, P. (1974), *Western Attitudes Toward Death: From the Middle Ages to the Present*, John Hopkins University Press.

Armstrong, D. (1987), 'Silence and truth in death and dying', *Social Science and Medicine*, 24, (8), pp. 651-657.

Ashby, D., Ames, D., West, C.R., Macdonald, A., Graham, N. and Mann, A. (1991), 'Psychiatric morbidity as a predictor of mortality for residents of local authority homes for the elderly', *International Journal Geriatric Psychiatry*, 6, pp. 567-575.

Baldwin, N., Harris, J. and Kelly, D. (1993), 'Institutionalisation: why blame the institution?', *Ageing and Society*, 13, pp. 69-81.

Becker, E. (1973), *The Denial of Death*, The Free Press.

Beier, L. (1989), *The Good Death in Seventeenth Century Britain*, London: Routledge.

Benoliel, J.Q. (1978), 'The changing social context for life and death decisions', *Essence*, 2, pp. 5-14.

Birley, M. F. (1960), 'Terminal care', *The Almoner*, 13, pp. 86-97.

Blauner, R. (1966), 'Death and social structure', *Psychiatry*, 29, pp. 378-394.

Bloch, M. and Parry, J. (1982), *Death and the Regeneration of Life*, Cambridge University Press.

Bond, J. and Bond S. (1994), *Sociology and Health Care*, Churchill Livingstone.

Booth, T. (1985), *Home Truths: Old People's Homes and the Outcomes of Care*, Gower.

Booth, T., Phillips, D., Barritt, A., Berry, S., Martin, D. and Melotte, C. (1983a), 'Patterns of mortality in homes for the elderly', *Age and Ageing*, 12, pp. 240-244.

Booth, T., Philips, D., Barritt, A., Berry, S., Martin, D. and Melotte, C. (1983b), 'A follow up study of trends in dependency in local authority homes for the elderly (1980-82)', *Research, Policy and Planning*, 1, no.1, pp. 1-9.

Bowlby, J. (1979), *The Making and Breaking of Affectional Bonds*, Social Science Paperbacks, Tavistock.

Brearley, P. C. (1981), *Residential Work with the Elderly*, Library of Social Work, Routledge and Kegan Paul.

Bromley, D. B. (1966), *The Psychology of Human Ageing*, Pelican.

Burritt, T. A., Berry, S., Martin, D.N. and Melotte, C. (1983), 'Dependency in residential homes for the elderly', *Social Policy and Administration*, 17, 2, pp. 46-62.

Butler, N. (1969), 'Ageism: another form of biology', *Gerontologist*, 9.

Butler, R. (1963), 'The life review: an interpretation of reminiscence in the aged', *Psychiatry*, 26, pp. 65-76.

Butler, R., and Lewis, M. (1973), *Aging and Mental Health*, St. Louis: C. V. Mosby Company.

Capon, L. J. (1956), *The Adams-Jefferson Letters*, University of North Carolina Press.

Cartwright, A. (1991), 'The role of residential and nursing homes in the last year of people's lives', *British Journal of Social Work*, 21, pp. 627-645.

Cartwright, A. and Seale, C.F. (1990), *The Natural History of a Survey: an Account of the Methodological Issues Encountered in a Study of Life before Death*, London: King's Fund.

Carse, J. P. (1980), *Death and Existence*, John Wiley & Sons.

Challis, D., Davies, B. and Traske, K. eds. (1994), *Community Care: New Agendas and Challenges for the UK and Overseas*, Arena Books/PSSRU, University of Kent.

Charlesworth, A. and Wilkin, D. (1982), *Dependency Among Old People in Geriatric Wards, Psycho-geriatric Wards and Residential Homes 1977-87, Research Report No 6*, University of Manchester Department of Psychiatry and Community Medicare.

Clark, D. ed. (1993), *The Future for Palliative Care Issues of Policy and Practice*, Open University Press.

Clarke, D. ed. (1993), *The Sociology of Death*, Blackwell.

Cole, T. R. (1992), *The Journey of Life - A Cultural History of Ageing in America*, Cambridge University Press.

Comfort, A. (1977), *A Good Age*, Beazley.

Cumming, E. and Henry, W. (1961), *Growing Old*, New York: Basic Books.

Dale, A., Evandrov, M., and Arber, S. (1987), 'The household structure of the elderly population in Britain', *Ageing and Society*, 7, pp. 37-56.

Davies, B. and Knapp, M. (1981), *Old People's Homes and the Production of Welfare*, Routledge & Kegan Paul.

Davitz, L. J. and Davitz, J. R. (1975), 'How do nurses feel when patients suffer?', *American Journal of Nursing*, 75, no.9.

De Beauvoir, S. (1972), *Old Age*, Penguin Books.

De Vries, R. G. (1981), 'Birth and death: social construction at the poles of existence', *Social Forces*, 59, pp. 1074-1093.

Dewey, M. E., Davidson, I. A. and Copeland, T. R. M. (1993), 'Expressed wish to die and mortality in older people: a community replication', *Age and Ageing*, 22, pp. 109 -113.

Dickenson, D. and Johnson, M. eds. (1993), *Death, Dying and Bereavement*, Sage Publications.

Dinnage, R. (1990), *The Ruffian on the Stair - Reflections on Death*, Penguin Books.

Downie, R. S. and Calman, K. C. (1987), *Healthy Respect*, London: Faber and Faber.

Durkheim, E. (1968), *Elementary Forms of Religious Life*, Paris: PUF.

Elias, N. (1985), *The Loneliness of the Dying*, Basil Blackwell.

Faden, R. R. and Beauchamp,T. L. (1986), *A History and Theory of Informed Consent*, New York: Oxford University Press.

Field, D. (1989), *Nursing the Dying*, London: Routledge & Kegan Paul.

Field, T. M., Huston, A., Quay, H. C., Troll, L. and Finley, G. E. eds. (1982), *Review of Human Development*, New York: Wiley.

Field, D. and James, N. (1993), 'Where and how people die' in *The Future of Palliative Care*, Clark, D. ed. Open University Press.

Finch, J. and Groves, D. eds. (1993), *A Labour of Love: Women, Work and Caring*, Routledge and Kegan Paul.

Finley, G. E. (1982), 'Modernisation and ageing', in Field, T. M., Huston, A., Quay, H. C., Troll, L. and Finley, eds. *Review of Human Development*, ch.15, pp. 511-523, New York: Wiley.

Fortune, R. (1932), *Sorcerers of Dobu: The Social Anthropology of the Dobu Islanders of the Western Pacific*, New York: Dutton.

Fowler, O. S. (1850), *Physiology: Animal and Mental*, New York: Fowlers and Wells.

Fox, N. J. (1993), *Postmodernity, Sociology and Health*, Open University Press.

Freud, S. (1917), 'Mourning and melancholia' in *Complete Psychological Works of Sigmund Freud*, Standard Edition, 14, Strachey, J. ed. New York: Norton.

Fries, J. and Crapo, L. (1981), *Vitality and Ageing*, San Francisco: Freeman.

Gilmore, A. and Gilmore, S. eds. (1988), *A Safer Death*, London: Plenum.

Glaser, B. G. and Strauss, A. L. (1965a), *Time for Dying*, Chicago: Aldine.

Glaser, B. G. and Strauss, A. L. (1965b), *Awareness of Dying*, Chicago:Aldine.

Glaser, B. G. and Strauss, A. L. (1967), *The Discovery of Grounded Theory: Strategies for Qualitative Research*, Chicago: Aldine.

Goffman, E. (1961), *Asylums: Essays on the Social Situation of Mental Patients and other Inmates*, Garden City, N.J: Anchor Books.

Goffman, E. (1964), *Stigma: Notes on the Management of Spoiled Identity*, Prentice-Hall.

Gorer, G. (1955), 'The pornography of death', *Encounter*, October.

Gorer, G. (1965), *Death, Grief and Mourning in Contemporary Britain*, Crescent Press.

Greenwood, E. (1966), 'The elements of professionalisation' in *Professionalisation*, Vollmer, H. M., and Mills, D. L. eds. Englewood-Cliffs: Prentice Hall.

Gubrium, J. F. and Sankar, A. eds. (1994), *Qualitative Methods in Aging Research*, Sage (Focus edition).

Habermas, J. (1974), *Theory and Practice*, Heinemann.

Hammersley, M. ed. (1993), *Social Research: Philosophy, Politics and Practice*, Sage.

Harrington, A. (1977), *The Immortalist*. Millbrace, Calif: Celestial Arts.

Heatherington, E. M. (1980), 'Children and divorce' in *Parents-Child Interaction*, Henderson, R. ed. Academic Press.

Hinton, J. (1972), *Dying*, Penguin Books.

Hockey, J. (1990), *Experiences of Death: an Anthropological Account*, Edinburgh University Press, Edinburgh.

Houlbrooke, R. ed. (1989), *Death, Ritual and Bereavement*, Routledge.

Howe, D. (1995), *Attachment Theory for Social Work Practice*, Macmillan.

Hughes, B. (1995), *Older People and Community Care: Critical Theory and Practice*, Open University Press.

James, V. (1986), *Care and Work in Nursing the Dying: A Participant Study of a Continuing Care Unit*, Unpublished PhD. thesis, University of Aberdeen.

Jones, K. and Fowles, A. J. (1984), *Ideas on Institutions*, Routledge and Kegan Paul.

Jones, S. (1985), 'Depth Interviewing' in *Applied Qualitative Research*, Walker, R. ed. Gower.

Kastenbaum, R., and Aisenberg, R. (1972), *The Psychology of Death*, New York: Springer.

Kearl, M. C. (1989), *Endings: A Sociology of Death and Dying*, Oxford University Press.

Kellehear, A. (1989), 'Are we a death denying society? A sociological review', *Social Science and Medicine*, 18, (9).

Klein, M. (1940), 'Mourning and its relationship to manic-depressive states', *International Journal of Psycho-Analysis*, 21, pp. 125-53.

Koestler, A. (1977), 'Cosmic Consciousness', *Psychology Today*,104, pp.53-4.

Kübler-Ross, E. (1970), *On Death and Dying*, London: Tavistock.

Lamerton, R. (1980), *Care of the Dying*, Penguin Books.

Larson, M. S. (1977), *The Rise of Professionalisation*, Berkeley: University of California Press.

Leonard, P. (1975), *Personality and Ideology: Towards a Materialist Understanding of the Individual*, London: Macmillan.

Lerner, M. (1970), 'When, why and where people die?' in *The Dying Patient*, Brim, O. G., Freeman, H. E. and Scotch, N. A. eds. New York: Russell Saye Foundation.

Lidz, C. W., Fischer, L. and Arnold, R. M. (1992), *The Erosion of Autonomy in Long-Term Care*, Oxford University Press.

Littlewood, J. (1992), *Aspects of Grief*, Routledge.

Lofland, L. (1978), *The Craft of Dying*, London: Sage.

Longman, P. (1987), *Born to Pay: The New Politics of Ageing America*, Boston: Houghton Mifflin.

Macdonald, A. J. D. and Dunn, G. (1982), 'Death and the expressed wish to die in the elderly: an outcome study', *Age and Ageing*, 11, pp. 189-195.

Marris, P. (1958), *Widows and their Families*, London: Routledge & Kegan Paul.

Marris, P. (1974), *Loss and Change*, London: Routledge & Kegan Paul.

Marshall, M. (1983), *Social Work with Old People*, London: Macmillan.

Martin, J. (1989), 'Doctor's mask on pain', *The Guardian*, (First Person).

Maxwell, F. S. (1968), *The Measure of my Days*, New York: Knopt.

Mellor, P. (1993), 'Death in high modernity: the contemporary presence and absence of death' in *The Sociology of Death*, Clarke, D. ed. Blackwell.

Miles, M. B. and Huberman, A. M. (1994), *Qualitative Data Analysis: An Expanded Sourcebook*, 2nd edition. Sage.

Miller, G. (1974), *Aberfan: A Disaster and its Aftermath*, London: Constable.

Murray-Parkes, C. (1988), 'Bereavement as a psycho-social transition: processes of adaptation to change', *Journal of Social Issues*, 44, pp. 53-65.

Murray-Parkes. C. (1972), *Bereavement*, London: Tavistock.

Pardi, M. M. (1977), *Death: An Anthropological Perspective*, University Press of America.

Payne, M. (1995), *Social Work and Community Care*, Macmillan.

Payne, R. and Firth-Cozens, J. eds. (1987), *Stress in Health Professions*, Chichester: John Wiley.

Peck, D. (1991), 'Towards a theory of suicide: the case for modern fatalism', *Omega*, 11 (1), pp. 1-14.

Perakyla, A. (1988), 'Four frames of death in the modern hospital' in *A Safer Death*, Gilmore, A. and Gilmore, S. eds. London: Plenum.

Pelling, M. and Smith, R. M. eds. (1991), *The Welfare of the Elderly in the Past*, Routledge.

Phillips, J. (1994), 'Working categories and frail older people' in *Community Care: New Agendas and Challenges for the UK and Overseas*, Challis, D., Davies, B. and Traske, K. eds. Arena Books/PSSRU, University of Kent.

Phillipson, C. (1986), 'The development of European social gerontology', *Ageing and Society*, 6, pp. 91-98.

Phillipson, C. and Walker, A. eds. (1986), *Ageing and Social Policy - A Critical Assessment*, Gower.

Pincus, L. (1974), *Death and the Family*, Faber and Faber.

Porter, C. S. (1842), *Abandonment of God Deprecated by the Aged*, Utica NY.

Poss, S. (1981), *Towards Death with Dignity*, Nat.Inst.Soc.Services, no.41, George Allen & Unwin.

Power, M., Clough, R., Gibson, P. and Kelly, S. (1993), *Helping Lively Minds: Volunteer Support in Residential Homes*, University of Bristol, School of Applied Social Studies.

Prior, L. (1989), *The Social Organisation of Death: Medical Discourse and Social Practices in Belfast*, London: MacMillan.

Qureshi, H. and Walker, A. (1989), *The Caring Relationship*. Macmillan.

Rackstraw, M. (1944), *An Old People's Hostel*, originally published in January by *Social Work* (London), reprinted by OPWC.

Radcliffe-Brown, A. R. (1922), *The Andaman Islanders*, Cambridge University Press.

Rosenblatt, P. C. (1983), *Bitter, Bitter Tears*, University of Minnesota Press.

Royal College of Nursing, (1992), *A Scandal Waiting to Happen? Elderly People and Nursing Care in Residential and Nursing Homes*, RCN.

Saunders, C. (1965), 'The last stages of life', *American Journal of Nursing*, 65, pp. 70-75.

Saunders, C. (1966), 'The concerns of the patient', *Contact*, 18 October, p. 13.

Seale, C. F. (1990), 'Caring for people who die', *Ageing and Society*, 10, pp. 413-428.

Seale, C. F. (1991), 'Death from cancer and death from other causes: the relevance of the hospice approach', *Palliative Medicine*, 5, pp. 12-19.

Seale, C. F. (1995), 'Dying Alone', *Sociology of Health and Illness*, 17, (3), pp. 376-392.

Shanfield, S. B. (1981), 'The mourning of the health care professional: an important element in education about death and loss', *Death Education*, 4, pp. 385-395.

Shilling, C. (1993), *The Body and Social Theory*, London: Sage.

Silverman, D. (1993), *Interpreting Qualitative Data: Methods for Analysing Talk, Text and Interaction*, Sage.

Singleton, R., Straits, B., Straits, M. and McAllister, R. (1988), *Approaches to Social Research*, Oxford University Press.

Smith, N. (1905), *Masters of Old Age*, Milwaukee: The Young Churchman.

Stedeford, A. (1984), *Facing Death. Patients, Families and Professionals*, Heinemann.

Stein, L. I., Watts, D. T. and Howell, T. (1990), 'The doctor-nurse game revisited', *New England Journal of Medicine*, 322, (8), pp. 546-549.

Stern, E. (1947), *Buried Alive*, Women's Home Companion.

Strachey, J. ed. (1957), *Complete Psychological Works of Sigmund Freud*, Standard Edition, New York: Norton.

Sudnow, D. (1967), *Passing On - A Social Organisation of Dying*, Prentice-Hall.

Tenenbaum, F. (1979), *Over 55 is not Illegal*, Boston: Houghton Mifflin.

Thompson, P. (1993), 'I don't feel old: subjective ageing and the search for meaning in later life', *Age and Ageing*, pp. 23-43.

Thomson, D. (1991), 'Life, death and the elderly: historical perspectives' in *The Welfare of the Elderly in the Past*, Pelling, M. and Smith, R.M. eds. Routledge.

Tobin, S, S. and Lieberman, M. A. (1976), *Last Home for the Aged: Critical Implications of Institutionalisation*, Jossey-Bass Limited.

Townsend, P. (1964), *The Last Refuge: A Survey of Residential Institutions and Homes for the Aged in England and Wales*, Routledge & Kegan Paul.

Twining, C. (1988), *Helping Older People - A Psychological Approach*, John Wiley & Sons.

Vachon, M. C. S. (1987), *Occupational Stress in Caring for the Chronically Ill, the Dying, and the Bereaved*, Washington DC: Hemisphere.

Van Maanen, J. (1979), 'The fact of fiction in organisational ethnography', *Administrative Science Quarterly*, 24, pp. 539-611.

Victor, C. R. (1987), *Old Age in Modern Society: A Textbook of Social Gerontology*, Chapman & Hall.

Wade, B. and Finlayson, J. (1983), 'Drugs and the elderly', *Nursing Mirror*, 4 May, pp. 17-21.

Walker, R. ed. (1985), *Applied Qualitative Research*, Gower.

Walter, T. (1992), 'Modern death: taboo or not taboo?' *Sociology*, 25 (2), pp. 293-310.

Wilkinson, S. (1991), 'Factors which influence how nurses communicate with cancer patients', *Journal of Advanced Nursing*, 1, (6), pp. 677-688.

Willcocks, D., Peace, S. and Kellaher, L. (1985), *Private Lives in Public Places*, London: Tavistock.

Williams, R. (1989) 'Awareness and control of dying: some paradoxical trends in public opinion', *Sociology of Health and Illness*, 3, pp. 201-212.

Wilson, G. (1939), 'Nyakyusa conventions of burial', *Bantu Studies*, 13, pp.1-31.

Zarit, S. H. (1978), *Readings in Ageing and Death: Contemporary Perspectives*, Harper and Row.

Author index

Tenenbaum 20
Thompson 10, 35
Thomson 9, 22
Tobin and Leiberman 99
Townsend 17, 22, 32, 33
Twining 33

Vachon 14, 28
Van Mannen 39

Victor 15, 16, 23, 26

Wade et al 27
Walter 7, 12, 29, 30, 35
Wilkinson 32
Willcocks et al 24, 26, 27
Wilson 32

Zarit 11, 15, 30